QUICK & EASY RENAL DIET COOKBOOK

Discover Effortless Renal-Friendly Recipes! Simplify Your Meal Planning, Enjoy Delicious Dishes Tailored For Kidney Health And Well-Being

Elizabeth Francis

Table of Contents

CHAPTER ONE 4

   Understanding Renal Diets 4

   Introduction to Renal Diets 4

   Importance of Diet in Renal Health 4

   Basics of a Renal Diet Plan 6

CHAPTER TWO 10

   Essential Nutrients for Renal Health 10

   Protein in Renal Diet 10

   Sodium Management 12

   Potassium and Phosphorus Balance 14

CHAPTER THREE 17

   Planning Your Renal Diet 17

   Meal Planning Strategies 17

   Grocery Shopping Tips 18

   Meal Prep for Renal Diets 20

CHAPTER FOUR 22

   Breakfast Delights 22

   Low-Potassium Pancakes and Waffles 22

Protein-Packed Smoothies 23

Oatmeal and Cereal Alternatives 25

CHAPTER FIVE 27

Lunchtime Favorites 27

Renal-Friendly Sandwiches and Wraps 27

Salads with Kidney-Friendly Dressings 28

Soups and Stews for Renal Diets 30

CHAPTER SIX 33

Dinner Creations 33

Flavorful Low-Sodium Entrees 33

Vegetarian Delights for Renal Diets 36

CHAPTER SEVEN 39

Snacks and Appetizers 39

Nutritious Renal-Friendly Snack Ideas 39

Appetizers for Renal Diet Restrictions 41

Homemade Salsas and Dips 43

CHAPTER EIGHT 46

Side Dishes and Accompaniments 46

Low-Phosphorus Vegetable Sides 46

Grain and Pasta Alternatives 47

Renal-Friendly Potato and Rice Dishes 49

CHAPTER NINE 52
Desserts and Treats 52
Fruit-Based Desserts with Low Potassium 52
Decadent Renal-Friendly Desserts 54
Sugar-Free and Low-Phosphorus Treats 56

CHAPTER TEN 59
Beverages and Drinks 59
Hydration Tips for Renal Health 59
Low-Potassium Drink Options 61
Homemade Infusions and Refreshing Beverages 63

CHAPTER ELEVEN 66
RENAL DIETS AND THEIR PREPARATION 66

THE END 115

COPYRIGHT © 2023

All rights reserved. No part of this publication may be reproduced, distributed, or transmitted in any form or by any means, including photocopying, recording, or other electronic or mechanical methods, without the prior written permission of the publisher, except in the case of brief quotations embodied in critical reviews and certain other noncommercial uses permitted by copyright law.

CHAPTER ONE

Understanding Renal Diets

Introduction to Renal Diets

Renal diets are specialized eating plans designed to support kidney health and manage conditions such as chronic kidney disease (CKD), kidney stones, and other kidney-related issues. These diets are tailored to manage the levels of certain nutrients that can affect kidney function, such as protein, potassium, phosphorus, and sodium. Understanding renal diets involves grasping the significance of these dietary modifications and their impact on overall kidney health.

Renal diets are not a one-size-fits-all approach; they are customized based on individual needs, stage of kidney disease, and other health factors. While a renal diet may seem restrictive, it plays a crucial role in slowing the progression of kidney disease, managing symptoms, and improving overall quality of life for those with kidney conditions.

Importance of Diet in Renal Health

Diet plays a pivotal role in maintaining optimal kidney health and managing kidney-related conditions. The kidneys are vital organs responsible for filtering waste products and excess fluids from the blood, regulating electrolyte balance, and producing hormones that help regulate blood pressure and red blood cell production. Certain dietary components can either support or strain kidney function, making dietary adjustments crucial for individuals with kidney issues.

1. **Managing Nutrient Levels**: Renal diets focus on controlling the intake of specific nutrients to alleviate stress on the kidneys. For instance, limiting protein intake reduces the burden on the kidneys by minimizing the production of waste products from protein metabolism. Similarly, controlling the intake of potassium, phosphorus, and sodium helps prevent imbalances that can exacerbate kidney disease.

2. **Blood Pressure Regulation**: High blood pressure is a common complication of kidney disease and can further damage the kidneys if left uncontrolled. A renal diet often includes strategies to lower sodium intake, as excess sodium can contribute to hypertension. Additionally, diets rich in fruits, vegetables, and whole grains provide nutrients that support blood pressure regulation and overall cardiovascular health.

3. **Managing Fluid Intake**: For individuals with compromised kidney function, regulating fluid intake is essential to prevent

fluid overload, which can strain the kidneys and lead to complications such as edema and high blood pressure. Renal diets typically include guidelines for monitoring and limiting fluid intake based on individual needs and stage of kidney disease.

4. **Preventing Complications**: Certain dietary factors can increase the risk of complications associated with kidney disease. For example, high phosphorus levels can contribute to bone disorders and cardiovascular complications, while excessive potassium intake can lead to dangerous heart rhythm abnormalities. By carefully managing nutrient intake through a renal diet, individuals can reduce the risk of these complications and improve overall health outcomes.

5. **Supporting Overall Health**: In addition to managing kidney-specific issues, renal diets aim to support overall health and well-being. This includes promoting a balanced intake of essential nutrients, maintaining a healthy weight, and preventing or managing comorbid conditions such as diabetes and cardiovascular disease. By addressing dietary factors that impact both kidney health and general health, renal diets contribute to a holistic approach to wellness.

Basics of a Renal Diet Plan

Designing a renal diet plan requires careful consideration of individual needs, medical history, stage of kidney disease, and dietary preferences. While specific recommendations may vary, there are general principles that guide the development of a renal diet plan:

1. **Protein Restriction**: Protein restriction is a cornerstone of renal diets, as excessive protein intake can increase the workload on the kidneys. Depending on the stage of kidney disease and individual factors, protein intake may be limited to prevent further kidney damage while ensuring adequate nutrition.

2. **Controlling Potassium Intake**: Potassium is a mineral that plays a crucial role in muscle function and heart health. However, elevated potassium levels can be dangerous for individuals with kidney disease, as impaired kidney function can lead to potassium buildup in the blood. Renal diets typically include recommendations for limiting high-potassium foods such as bananas, oranges, tomatoes, and potatoes.

3. **Managing Phosphorus Levels**: Phosphorus is another mineral that requires careful monitoring in renal diets. Elevated phosphorus levels can contribute to bone disorders and cardiovascular complications. To manage phosphorus intake, individuals may be advised to limit foods high in phosphorus, such as dairy products, nuts, seeds, and processed foods containing phosphate additives.

4. **Limiting Sodium Intake**: Sodium restriction is essential for managing blood pressure and fluid balance in individuals with kidney disease. Renal diets often emphasize reducing the consumption of high-sodium foods such as processed meats, canned soups, and salty snacks. Instead, individuals are encouraged to flavor foods with herbs, spices, and other low-sodium alternatives.

5. **Monitoring Fluid Intake**: Regulating fluid intake is crucial for individuals with kidney disease, especially those experiencing fluid retention or swelling. Renal diets may include guidelines for monitoring fluid intake and adjusting consumption based on individual needs and recommendations from healthcare providers.

6. **Individualized Approach**: Renal diet plans should be individualized to meet the unique needs and preferences of each person. Factors such as age, gender, activity level, comorbid conditions, and cultural dietary practices should be taken into account when designing a renal diet plan. Regular monitoring and adjustments may be necessary to ensure optimal nutrition and kidney health.

In conclusion, understanding renal diets involves recognizing the importance of dietary modifications in supporting kidney health and managing kidney-related conditions. Renal diets aim to optimize nutrient intake while minimizing the burden on the kidneys, promoting overall health and well-being for individuals with kidney disease. By following the basics of a renal diet plan and working closely with healthcare providers and registered dietitians, individuals can effectively manage their condition and improve their quality of life.

CHAPTER TWO

Essential Nutrients for Renal Health

Maintaining optimal renal health involves careful management of essential nutrients to support kidney function and prevent complications associated with kidney disease. Protein, sodium, potassium, and phosphorus are among the key nutrients that require attention in renal diets. Understanding their roles and the strategies for managing them is essential for individuals with kidney conditions.

Protein in Renal Diet

Protein is a vital macronutrient necessary for building and repairing tissues, synthesizing hormones and enzymes, and supporting immune function. However, excessive protein intake can strain the kidneys, particularly in individuals with compromised kidney function. Therefore, protein management is a crucial aspect of renal diets.

1. **Protein Restriction**: In the early stages of kidney disease, protein restriction may not be necessary. However, as kidney function declines, reducing protein intake becomes

important to lessen the workload on the kidneys. High-protein diets can increase the production of waste products, such as urea and creatinine, which must be filtered by the kidneys. By moderating protein intake, individuals can slow the progression of kidney disease and minimize the risk of complications.

2. **Quality vs. Quantity**: When restricting protein intake, the focus shifts from quantity to quality. Instead of consuming large amounts of protein, individuals are encouraged to prioritize high-quality protein sources that provide essential amino acids without excessive waste products. Examples of high-quality protein sources include lean meats, poultry, fish, eggs, dairy products, and plant-based sources such as legumes, tofu, and nuts.

3. **Individualized Recommendations**: Protein intake recommendations in renal diets are tailored to individual needs, taking into account factors such as age, gender, stage of kidney disease, nutritional status, and activity level. Registered dietitians work with individuals to determine the appropriate level of protein intake to meet nutritional needs while minimizing strain on the kidneys.

4. **Supervised Monitoring**: Regular monitoring of protein intake and kidney function is essential for individuals following a renal diet. Healthcare providers and dietitians monitor blood

urea nitrogen (BUN) and serum creatinine levels to assess kidney function and ensure that protein intake is appropriate for individual needs and disease progression.

Overall, protein management plays a critical role in renal diets, balancing the need for essential nutrients with the requirement to minimize stress on the kidneys. By focusing on high-quality protein sources and individualized recommendations, individuals can support kidney health and optimize nutritional status.

Sodium Management

Sodium, a mineral found in salt and many processed foods, plays a significant role in fluid balance, nerve function, and muscle contraction. However, excessive sodium intake can contribute to high blood pressure, fluid retention, and cardiovascular complications, making sodium management an essential aspect of renal diets.

1. **Impact of Sodium on Kidney Health**: Excess sodium can impair kidney function by increasing blood pressure and promoting fluid retention. In individuals with kidney disease, the kidneys may struggle to excrete excess sodium, leading to further complications. Therefore, sodium restriction is crucial for managing blood pressure and fluid balance in renal diets.

2. **Sodium Restriction Guidelines**: Renal diets typically include guidelines for limiting sodium intake to reduce the risk of

complications. The recommended daily sodium intake varies depending on individual factors such as age, kidney function, and presence of other health conditions. However, most renal diet plans advise keeping sodium intake below 2,300 milligrams per day, with further restrictions for those with more advanced kidney disease or hypertension.

3. **Sources of Dietary Sodium**: Sodium is abundant in processed and packaged foods, as well as restaurant meals and fast food. Common sources of dietary sodium include canned soups, processed meats, snack foods, condiments, and prepared sauces. Reading food labels and choosing low-sodium alternatives can help individuals reduce their sodium intake while still enjoying flavorful meals.

4. **Tips for Sodium Reduction**: Renal diet plans often include practical tips for reducing sodium intake while maintaining flavor and variety in the diet. These may include cooking at home using fresh ingredients, seasoning foods with herbs and spices instead of salt, rinsing canned vegetables to remove excess sodium, and avoiding high-sodium condiments and sauces.

5. **Fluid Balance Considerations**: Sodium management is closely linked to fluid balance in renal diets. Excess sodium can lead to fluid retention, exacerbating swelling and increasing the risk of hypertension and cardiovascular

complications. By reducing sodium intake and maintaining a healthy fluid balance, individuals can support kidney function and overall health.

In conclusion, sodium management is a critical component of renal diets, supporting kidney health and reducing the risk of complications associated with kidney disease. By following guidelines for sodium restriction and making informed food choices, individuals can optimize their nutritional intake while protecting their kidneys.

Potassium and Phosphorus Balance

Potassium and phosphorus are essential minerals that play vital roles in various physiological processes, including nerve function, muscle contraction, and bone health. However, imbalances in potassium and phosphorus levels can have significant implications for individuals with kidney disease, making careful management of these nutrients essential in renal diets.

1. **Potassium Regulation**: Potassium is primarily excreted by the kidneys, so impaired kidney function can lead to potassium buildup in the blood, a condition known as hyperkalemia. High potassium levels can disrupt normal heart rhythm and increase the risk of cardiovascular complications. Therefore, potassium regulation is a key focus of renal diets.

2. **High-Potassium Foods**: Potassium-rich foods include fruits, vegetables, dairy products, nuts, seeds, and legumes. While these foods are nutritious, individuals with kidney disease may need to limit their intake to avoid elevated potassium levels. Renal diet plans often provide guidelines for identifying and moderating consumption of high-potassium foods based on individual needs and kidney function.

3. **Phosphorus Management**: Phosphorus is a mineral found in many foods, particularly protein-rich foods, dairy products, nuts, and whole grains. In individuals with kidney disease, impaired kidney function can lead to phosphorus retention and elevated phosphorus levels in the blood, a condition known as hyperphosphatemia. High phosphorus levels can contribute to bone disorders, cardiovascular complications, and other health issues.

4. **Phosphorus Binders**: In addition to dietary restrictions, some individuals with advanced kidney disease may require phosphorus binders to help control phosphorus levels. These medications bind to dietary phosphorus in the gastrointestinal tract, preventing its absorption and reducing phosphorus levels in the blood. Phosphorus binders are typically taken with meals and snacks as prescribed by healthcare providers.

5. **Balancing Nutritional Needs**: Balancing potassium and phosphorus restrictions with nutritional requirements is a key consideration in renal diets. While it is important to limit high-potassium and high-phosphorus foods, individuals still need to obtain essential nutrients from other sources. Registered dietitians work with individuals to develop personalized meal plans that meet nutritional needs while minimizing the risk of complications associated with kidney disease.

6. **Supervised Monitoring**: Regular monitoring of potassium and phosphorus levels is essential for individuals following renal diets. Healthcare providers monitor blood tests to assess electrolyte balance and kidney function, making adjustments to dietary recommendations as needed to maintain optimal health.

In summary, potassium and phosphorus balance are critical components of renal diets, supporting kidney health and reducing the risk of complications associated with kidney disease. By following guidelines for potassium and phosphorus regulation and working closely with healthcare providers and dietitians, individuals can optimize their nutritional intake and support overall kidney function.

CHAPTER THREE

Planning Your Renal Diet

Planning a renal diet involves careful consideration of nutrient restrictions, individual dietary preferences, and practical strategies for meal preparation and grocery shopping. By incorporating meal planning strategies, grocery shopping tips, and meal prep techniques tailored to renal diets, individuals can effectively manage their condition while enjoying delicious and nutritious meals.

Meal Planning Strategies

Meal planning is a fundamental aspect of a renal diet, helping individuals adhere to nutrient restrictions while ensuring balanced and flavorful meals. Here are some strategies for effective meal planning:

1. **Focus on Nutrient Balance**: When planning meals for a renal diet, prioritize nutrient balance by incorporating a variety of foods from different food groups. Aim to include lean protein sources, whole grains, fruits, vegetables, and healthy

fats in each meal to ensure adequate nutrition while meeting dietary restrictions.

2. **Portion Control**: Pay attention to portion sizes when planning meals, especially when it comes to protein-rich foods and high-potassium or high-phosphorus items. Use measuring cups, scales, or visual cues to portion out appropriate serving sizes and avoid overconsumption of restricted nutrients.

3. **Incorporate Variety**: Keep meals interesting and enjoyable by incorporating a variety of flavors, textures, and cooking methods. Experiment with different recipes, spices, and cooking techniques to add variety to your meals while adhering to renal diet guidelines.

4. **Plan Ahead for Special Occasions**: Consider special occasions or events when planning meals to accommodate dietary restrictions while still enjoying celebratory foods. Look for renal-friendly recipes or adapt traditional dishes to meet your nutritional needs without compromising on taste.

5. **Consult with a Dietitian**: If you're unsure about how to plan meals that meet your specific dietary needs, consult with a registered dietitian who specializes in renal nutrition. A dietitian can provide personalized guidance and meal planning support based on your individual health status, preferences, and goals.

Grocery Shopping Tips

Navigating the grocery store can be challenging when following a renal diet, but with some helpful tips, you can make informed choices and select foods that align with your nutritional requirements:

1. **Read Food Labels**: Become familiar with reading food labels to identify hidden sources of sodium, potassium, and phosphorus in packaged foods. Pay attention to serving sizes, nutrient content, and ingredient lists to make informed choices.

2. **Choose Fresh, Whole Foods**: Focus on purchasing fresh, whole foods such as fruits, vegetables, lean meats, poultry, fish, and whole grains. These foods are typically lower in sodium and phosphorus and can be incorporated into a renal-friendly diet with ease.

3. **Limit Processed and Packaged Foods**: Minimize your intake of processed and packaged foods, as they often contain high levels of sodium, phosphorus additives, and other potentially harmful ingredients. Opt for fresh or frozen alternatives whenever possible.

4. **Stock Up on Renal-Friendly Staples**: Keep your pantry stocked with renal-friendly staples such as low-sodium broths, canned fruits in juice (rather than syrup), dried herbs and spices (instead of seasoning blends containing salt),

whole grain pasta and rice, and canned beans (rinsed to reduce sodium content).

5. **Shop the Perimeter of the Store**: The perimeter of the grocery store typically contains fresh produce, meats, dairy products, and other whole foods, while the inner aisles often house processed and packaged items. Focus on shopping the perimeter to prioritize nutrient-dense, renal-friendly foods.

Meal Prep for Renal Diets

Meal prep can streamline the cooking process and make it easier to adhere to a renal diet, especially on busy days. Here are some meal prep tips for renal diets:

1. **Plan Your Meals in Advance**: Take some time at the beginning of each week to plan your meals for the upcoming days. Consider your schedule, nutritional needs, and preferences when selecting recipes and preparing your grocery list.

2. **Batch Cook Protein**: Cook large batches of lean protein sources such as chicken breast, turkey, or fish at once, then portion them out and store them in the refrigerator or freezer for easy access throughout the week. Incorporate cooked protein into salads, wraps, stir-fries, and other dishes for quick and convenient meals.

3. **Prep Fruits and Vegetables**: Wash, chop, and portion out fruits and vegetables in advance to make it easier to incorporate them into meals and snacks. Store prepped produce in airtight containers or resealable bags in the refrigerator for maximum freshness and convenience.

4. **Cook Whole Grains in Bulk**: Prepare whole grains such as brown rice, quinoa, or barley in large batches and portion them out for use in salads, soups, grain bowls, and other dishes throughout the week. Cooked grains can be stored in the refrigerator or freezer and reheated as needed.

5. **Utilize Slow Cookers and Instant Pots**: Slow cookers and Instant Pots are invaluable tools for batch cooking and meal prep. Use them to prepare hearty stews, soups, chili, and other one-pot meals that can be portioned out and enjoyed over several days.

By incorporating these meal planning strategies, grocery shopping tips, and meal prep techniques into your routine, you can successfully navigate a renal diet and support your kidney health while enjoying delicious and nutritious meals. Remember to consult with a healthcare provider or registered dietitian for personalized guidance and support tailored to your individual needs and goals.

CHAPTER FOUR

Breakfast Delights

Breakfast is often considered the most important meal of the day, providing essential nutrients and energy to kick-start your morning. For individuals following a renal diet, breakfast can still be delicious and satisfying with the right recipes and choices. Here are some breakfast delights tailored to renal diets:

Low-Potassium Pancakes and Waffles

Pancakes and waffles are classic breakfast favorites that can be modified to meet the dietary restrictions of a renal diet. By using low-potassium ingredients and limiting the use of high-potassium toppings, you can enjoy these breakfast treats without compromising your kidney health.

1. **Ingredient Modifications**: Substitute traditional pancake and waffle ingredients with low-potassium alternatives. Use white flour or a combination of white and whole wheat flour instead of whole wheat flour, which is higher in potassium.

Replace milk with a low-potassium milk alternative such as rice milk or almond milk, and use baking powder instead of baking soda to minimize potassium content.

2. **Topping Choices**: Be mindful of topping choices to keep potassium levels in check. Instead of high-potassium fruits like bananas or oranges, opt for lower-potassium options such as strawberries, blueberries, or raspberries. You can also enjoy toppings such as whipped cream, sugar-free syrup, or a sprinkle of powdered sugar for added flavor without increasing potassium intake.

3. **Portion Control**: Pay attention to portion sizes when enjoying pancakes and waffles, especially if you have specific dietary restrictions or are monitoring your carbohydrate intake. Consider using a smaller-sized waffle iron or portioning out smaller servings of pancake batter to help control portion sizes and prevent overconsumption.

4. **Recipe Adaptations**: Look for renal-friendly pancake and waffle recipes that have been specifically modified to meet the nutritional needs of individuals with kidney disease. These recipes often use alternative ingredients and portion sizes to ensure they are suitable for a renal diet while still being delicious and satisfying.

Protein-Packed Smoothies

Smoothies are a convenient and nutritious option for breakfast, providing a quick and easy way to incorporate protein, fruits, and vegetables into your morning routine. By choosing kidney-friendly ingredients and avoiding high-potassium additions, you can create protein-packed smoothies that support your renal health.

1. **Protein Sources**: Include protein-rich ingredients such as low-potassium protein powders, Greek yogurt, silken tofu, or pasteurized liquid egg whites in your smoothies to boost protein content without increasing potassium levels. You can also add nut butters such as almond butter or peanut butter for added protein and flavor.

2. **Low-Potassium Fruits and Vegetables**: Select low-potassium fruits and vegetables as smoothie ingredients to keep potassium levels in check. Good options include berries (such as strawberries, blueberries, or raspberries), apples, pears, spinach, kale, cucumber, and celery. Be cautious with high-potassium fruits like bananas and oranges, and use them sparingly or avoid them altogether.

3. **Liquid Base**: Choose a low-potassium liquid base for your smoothies, such as water, rice milk, almond milk, or coconut water. Avoid using dairy milk or high-potassium fruit juices, as they can significantly increase the potassium content of your smoothie.

4. **Flavor Enhancements**: Add flavor to your smoothies with ingredients such as vanilla extract, cocoa powder, cinnamon, or fresh herbs like mint or basil. These flavor enhancers can help make your smoothie more enjoyable without adding unnecessary potassium.

5. **Portion Control**: Be mindful of portion sizes when enjoying smoothies, as they can be calorie-dense and high in carbohydrates if not consumed in moderation. Aim for a balanced combination of protein, fruits, and vegetables in each smoothie, and consider splitting larger servings into smaller portions to help manage your nutrient intake.

Oatmeal and Cereal Alternatives

Oatmeal and cereal are breakfast staples that can be modified to fit a renal diet by choosing low-potassium options and making strategic ingredient substitutions. With the right choices, you can enjoy a hearty and satisfying breakfast without compromising your kidney health.

1. **Low-Potassium Grain Choices**: Opt for low-potassium grains such as rolled oats, cream of wheat, or rice cereal as the base for your breakfast bowl. These grains are lower in potassium compared to alternatives like whole wheat or bran cereals, making them suitable options for individuals with kidney disease.

2. **Liquid Options**: Use low-potassium liquids such as water, rice milk, almond milk, or coconut milk to cook your oatmeal or cereal instead of traditional dairy milk. These alternatives provide moisture and flavor without adding significant amounts of potassium.

3. **Toppings and Add-Ins**: Choose kidney-friendly toppings and add-ins to enhance the flavor and nutritional content of your oatmeal or cereal. Options include sliced apples, pears, or berries; chopped nuts or seeds (such as almonds, walnuts, or chia seeds); and flavorings such as cinnamon, nutmeg, or vanilla extract.

4. **Portion Control**: Pay attention to portion sizes when preparing oatmeal or cereal to avoid excessive calorie and carbohydrate intake. Use measuring cups or kitchen scales to portion out appropriate serving sizes, and consider adding protein-rich ingredients such as Greek yogurt or nut butter to help balance your meal.

5. **Recipe Variations**: Experiment with different oatmeal and cereal recipes to keep breakfast interesting and varied. Try overnight oats, baked oatmeal squares, or savory oatmeal bowls with toppings like avocado, eggs, and salsa for a twist on traditional breakfast options.

By incorporating these breakfast delights into your renal diet, you can start your day on a nutritious and delicious note while supporting your kidney health. Remember to consult with a healthcare provider or registered dietitian for personalized guidance and recommendations tailored to your individual dietary needs and preferences.

CHAPTER FIVE

Lunchtime Favorites

Lunch is an important meal that provides energy and sustenance to fuel the rest of the day. For individuals following a renal diet, it's essential to choose lunch options that are both delicious and kidney-friendly. Here are some lunchtime favorites tailored to renal diets:

Renal-Friendly Sandwiches and Wraps

Sandwiches and wraps are versatile lunch options that can be customized to meet the dietary restrictions of a renal diet. By selecting low-potassium ingredients and using whole grain bread or wraps, you can enjoy a satisfying and nutritious meal without compromising your kidney health.

1. **Bread and Wrap Choices**: Opt for whole grain bread or wraps as the base for your sandwich or wrap. Whole grains are lower in potassium compared to refined grains and provide additional fiber and nutrients. Look for options labeled "whole grain" or "whole wheat" on the packaging to ensure you're making a kidney-friendly choice.

2. **Protein Sources**: Choose lean protein sources such as skinless chicken breast, turkey, tuna, or tofu to fill your sandwich or wrap. These protein options are lower in potassium compared to processed meats like deli ham or roast beef and provide essential nutrients without excessive sodium or phosphorus.

3. **Vegetable Fillings**: Load up your sandwich or wrap with kidney-friendly vegetables such as lettuce, spinach, cucumbers, bell peppers, and tomatoes. These vegetables are low in potassium and add texture, flavor, and nutrition to your meal. Be cautious with high-potassium vegetables like avocado and potatoes, and use them sparingly if desired.

4. **Condiments and Spreads**: Choose low-potassium condiments and spreads to enhance the flavor of your sandwich or wrap. Options include mustard, hummus, salsa, or low-sodium mayonnaise. Be mindful of high-potassium condiments like ketchup and barbecue sauce, and use them sparingly or avoid them altogether.

5. **Portion Control**: Pay attention to portion sizes when assembling your sandwich or wrap to avoid excessive calorie and sodium intake. Use measuring cups or visual cues to portion out appropriate amounts of ingredients, and aim for a balanced combination of protein, vegetables, and whole grains in each serving.

Salads with Kidney-Friendly Dressings

Salads are a refreshing and nutritious lunch option that can be adapted to fit a renal diet by choosing kidney-friendly ingredients and dressings. By incorporating low-potassium vegetables, lean protein sources, and homemade dressings, you can enjoy a satisfying salad that supports your kidney health.

1. **Leafy Greens**: Start with a base of leafy greens such as spinach, kale, or mixed salad greens. These greens are low in potassium and provide essential vitamins, minerals, and fiber to support overall health. Avoid high-potassium greens like Swiss chard and beet greens, and opt for lower-potassium alternatives instead.

2. **Protein Additions**: Add lean protein sources to your salad to make it more filling and satisfying. Options include grilled chicken breast, hard-boiled eggs, canned tuna or salmon, tofu, or cooked beans such as chickpeas or black beans. These protein sources are lower in potassium compared to

processed meats and provide essential nutrients without excessive sodium or phosphorus.

3. **Kidney-Friendly Vegetables**: Incorporate kidney-friendly vegetables into your salad for added flavor and nutrition. Good options include cucumbers, bell peppers, carrots, radishes, and cherry tomatoes. These vegetables are low in potassium and add texture and color to your salad without compromising your kidney health.

4. **Homemade Dressings**: Make your own kidney-friendly dressings using low-potassium ingredients such as olive oil, vinegar, lemon juice, herbs, and spices. Avoid store-bought dressings, which may contain high levels of sodium, phosphorus additives, and other potentially harmful ingredients. Homemade dressings allow you to control the ingredients and customize the flavor to suit your preferences.

5. **Toppings and Add-Ins**: Enhance the flavor and texture of your salad with kidney-friendly toppings and add-ins. Options include chopped nuts or seeds (such as almonds, walnuts, or sunflower seeds), dried cranberries or raisins, crumbled feta or goat cheese (in moderation), and avocado (used sparingly). Be mindful of portion sizes and choose toppings that align with your dietary restrictions.

Soups and Stews for Renal Diets

Soups and stews are hearty and comforting lunch options that can be adapted to fit a renal diet by selecting kidney-friendly ingredients and limiting the use of high-potassium additions. By making homemade versions with low-potassium vegetables, lean protein sources, and homemade broths, you can enjoy a nutritious and delicious meal that supports your kidney health.

1. **Broth-Based Soups**: Start with a base of low-sodium broth or stock for your soup or stew. Homemade broths allow you to control the sodium content and avoid excessive potassium additives found in many store-bought options. Choose chicken, vegetable, or beef broth labeled as "low-sodium" or "reduced sodium" for the best results.

2. **Lean Protein Sources**: Add lean protein sources to your soup or stew to make it more filling and nutritious. Options include skinless chicken breast, turkey, lean cuts of beef or pork, tofu, or legumes such as lentils or beans. These protein sources are lower in potassium compared to processed meats and provide essential nutrients without excessive sodium or phosphorus.

3. **Kidney-Friendly Vegetables**: Incorporate kidney-friendly vegetables into your soup or stew for added flavor and nutrition. Good options include onions, carrots, celery, bell peppers, zucchini, and spinach. These vegetables are low in

potassium and add texture and color to your dish without compromising your kidney health.

4. **Seasonings and Flavorings**: Use herbs, spices, and seasonings to enhance the flavor of your soup or stew without adding extra sodium or potassium. Options include garlic, onion powder, black pepper, thyme, rosemary, and bay leaves. Experiment with different combinations to create delicious and satisfying meals that meet your dietary restrictions.

5. **Portion Control**: Pay attention to portion sizes when serving soup or stew to avoid excessive calorie and sodium intake. Use measuring cups or kitchen scales to portion out appropriate serving sizes, and aim for a balanced combination of broth, protein, vegetables, and grains or legumes in each serving.

By incorporating these lunchtime favorites into your renal diet, you can enjoy delicious and satisfying meals that support your kidney health and overall well-being. Remember to consult with a healthcare provider or registered dietitian for personalized guidance and recommendations tailored to your individual dietary needs and preferences.

CHAPTER SIX

Dinner Creations

Dinner is an opportunity to enjoy a satisfying and flavorful meal while adhering to the dietary restrictions of a renal diet. By selecting kidney-friendly ingredients and preparing delicious entrees, you can create dinner creations that support your kidney health and satisfy your taste buds. Here are some dinner ideas tailored to renal diets:

Flavorful Low-Sodium Entrees

Entrees are the centerpiece of any dinner, and with the right ingredients and seasonings, you can create flavorful low-sodium options that are suitable for a renal diet. By using herbs, spices, and other flavor enhancers, you can elevate the taste of your dishes without relying on excessive salt.

1. **Herbs and Spices**: Experiment with a variety of herbs and spices to add flavor to your entrees without increasing sodium intake. Options include garlic, onion powder, black pepper, paprika, cumin, oregano, thyme, rosemary, and basil. Fresh herbs like parsley, cilantro, and chives can also add freshness and aroma to your dishes.

2. **Citrus**: Use citrus fruits such as lemon, lime, and orange to add brightness and acidity to your entrees. Citrus zest and juice can enhance the flavor of meats, poultry, fish, and vegetables without adding extra sodium. Consider using citrus marinades or sauces to infuse your dishes with vibrant flavor.

3. **Vinegar**: Incorporate vinegar into your cooking to add tanginess and depth of flavor to your entrees. Options include balsamic vinegar, apple cider vinegar, red wine vinegar, and rice vinegar. Vinegar-based marinades, dressings, and sauces can help tenderize meats and add complexity to your dishes.

4. **Homemade Sauces and Condiments**: Make your own sauces and condiments using low-sodium ingredients and flavorings. Options include homemade tomato sauce, salsa,

pesto, tzatziki, and chimichurri. These homemade creations allow you to control the sodium content and customize the flavor to suit your preferences.

5. **Roasting and Grilling**: Use roasting and grilling techniques to enhance the natural flavors of your ingredients. Roasting vegetables and meats caramelizes their sugars and intensifies their flavor, while grilling adds smokiness and charred notes. Experiment with different cooking methods to create delicious and memorable entrees.

Grilled and Baked Fish Options

Fish is a nutritious and kidney-friendly protein option that can be prepared in a variety of ways to suit your taste preferences. Grilling and baking are healthy cooking methods that preserve the natural flavors of fish while minimizing added fats and sodium.

1. **Lean and Mild Fish**: Choose lean and mild-flavored fish varieties that are suitable for renal diets. Good options include tilapia, cod, halibut, haddock, sole, flounder, and catfish. These fish varieties are lower in potassium and phosphorus compared to fattier fish like salmon and trout.

2. **Simple Seasonings**: Season fish with a combination of herbs, spices, and citrus to enhance its natural flavor without adding extra sodium. Options include lemon pepper seasoning, garlic and herb seasoning, Cajun seasoning, and

fresh herbs like dill, parsley, and chives. Brush fish with olive oil or a low-sodium marinade before grilling or baking to keep it moist and flavorful.

3. **Grilling Techniques**: Preheat your grill to medium-high heat and lightly oil the grates to prevent sticking. Place fish fillets or steaks directly on the grill and cook for a few minutes on each side until they are opaque and flake easily with a fork. Avoid overcooking fish to prevent it from becoming dry and tough.

4. **Baking Methods**: Preheat your oven to the desired temperature and line a baking sheet with parchment paper or aluminum foil for easy cleanup. Place fish fillets or steaks on the prepared baking sheet and season them with your chosen herbs and spices. Bake in the oven until the fish is cooked through and flakes easily with a fork.

5. **Serving Suggestions**: Serve grilled or baked fish with kidney-friendly side dishes such as roasted vegetables, steamed greens, quinoa, or brown rice. Garnish fish with fresh herbs, lemon wedges, or a drizzle of homemade sauce or dressing for added flavor and visual appeal.

Vegetarian Delights for Renal Diets

Vegetarian meals can be delicious, nutritious, and kidney-friendly when prepared with wholesome ingredients and balanced flavors. By incorporating plant-based protein sources, whole grains, and kidney-friendly vegetables, you can create vegetarian delights that are both satisfying and supportive of your kidney health.

1. **Plant-Based Protein Sources**: Include plant-based protein sources such as beans, lentils, tofu, tempeh, and edamame in your vegetarian meals to provide essential nutrients and promote satiety. These protein options are lower in potassium and phosphorus compared to animal proteins and offer a variety of textures and flavors to your dishes.

2. **Whole Grains**: Incorporate whole grains such as quinoa, brown rice, barley, farro, and bulgur into your vegetarian meals to add fiber, vitamins, and minerals. Whole grains are lower in potassium and phosphorus compared to refined grains and provide sustained energy to keep you feeling satisfied.

3. **Kidney-Friendly Vegetables**: Choose kidney-friendly vegetables such as leafy greens, bell peppers, cucumbers, carrots, and zucchini to add color, flavor, and nutrition to your vegetarian dishes. These vegetables are low in potassium and can be enjoyed in salads, stir-fries, soups, and casseroles.

4. **Flavorful Sauces and Dressings**: Use flavorful sauces and dressings to enhance the taste of your vegetarian dishes without relying on excessive sodium. Options include tahini

sauce, pesto, salsa, curry sauce, peanut sauce, and homemade vinaigrettes made with low-sodium ingredients. Experiment with different flavor combinations to create unique and satisfying meals.

5. **Creative Cooking Techniques**: Get creative with your cooking techniques to make vegetarian meals more exciting and appealing. Try grilling or roasting vegetables to bring out their natural sweetness, sautéing tofu or tempeh with aromatic spices and herbs, or simmering beans and lentils in flavorful broths and sauces. These techniques can elevate the taste and texture of your vegetarian dishes and make them more enjoyable to eat.

By incorporating these dinner creations into your renal diet, you can enjoy delicious and satisfying meals that support your kidney health and overall well-being. Remember to consult with a healthcare provider or registered dietitian for personalized guidance and recommendations tailored to your individual dietary needs and preferences.

CHAPTER SEVEN

Snacks and Appetizers

Snacks and appetizers are an integral part of any diet, providing a convenient and enjoyable way to satisfy hunger between meals or kick off a gathering. For individuals following a renal diet, choosing kidney-friendly options is essential to support overall health. Here are some ideas for nutritious snacks and appetizers tailored to renal diets:

Nutritious Renal-Friendly Snack Ideas

Snacking can be an opportunity to incorporate additional nutrients into your diet while keeping hunger at bay. By choosing kidney-friendly snack options that are low in potassium, sodium, and phosphorus, you can support your kidney health and maintain overall well-being. Here are some nutritious snack ideas for individuals with renal restrictions:

1. **Fresh Fruit**: Enjoy fresh fruits that are low in potassium, such as apples, berries (strawberries, blueberries, raspberries), grapes, and pineapple. These fruits provide natural sweetness and fiber while keeping potassium intake in check.

2. **Vegetable Sticks**: Cut up crunchy vegetables like carrots, celery, bell peppers, and cucumber into sticks or slices for a refreshing and low-potassium snack. Pair them with a kidney-friendly dip or hummus for added flavor and protein.

3. **Nuts and Seeds**: Snack on small portions of unsalted nuts and seeds, such as almonds, walnuts, pumpkin seeds, or sunflower seeds. These nutrient-dense snacks provide healthy fats, protein, and fiber to keep you feeling satisfied between meals.

4. **Greek Yogurt**: Choose low-fat or non-fat Greek yogurt as a protein-rich snack option. Greek yogurt is lower in potassium and phosphorus compared to regular yogurt and can be enjoyed plain or with a sprinkle of cinnamon or a drizzle of honey for added flavor.

5. **Rice Cakes with Nut Butter**: Spread a thin layer of unsalted nut butter (such as almond or cashew butter) onto a rice cake for a crunchy and satisfying snack. Rice cakes are low in potassium and provide a neutral base for your favorite nut butter.

6. **Hard-Boiled Eggs**: Hard-boiled eggs are a convenient and protein-packed snack that can be enjoyed on their own or sliced and added to salads or sandwiches. They provide essential nutrients like protein, vitamins, and minerals while being low in potassium and phosphorus.

7. **Cottage Cheese with Fruit**: Enjoy a small serving of low-fat cottage cheese with sliced fruit such as peaches, melon, or kiwi for a refreshing and protein-rich snack. Cottage cheese is lower in potassium compared to other dairy products and provides calcium and protein for bone and muscle health.

8. **Popcorn**: Air-popped popcorn is a satisfying and low-potassium snack option that can be enjoyed in moderation. Skip the added butter and salt and season your popcorn with herbs, spices, or nutritional yeast for extra flavor without increasing sodium intake.

Appetizers for Renal Diet Restrictions

Appetizers are a great way to start a meal or social gathering, and with the right ingredients, you can create kidney-friendly options that are both delicious and nutritious. By choosing appetizers that are low in sodium, potassium, and phosphorus, you can support your kidney health and enjoy guilt-free indulgence. Here are some appetizer ideas for individuals with renal diet restrictions:

1. **Fresh Vegetable Platter**: Create a colorful vegetable platter with an assortment of kidney-friendly vegetables such as

cherry tomatoes, cucumber slices, carrot sticks, bell pepper strips, and snap peas. Serve with a low-sodium dip or hummus for added flavor and protein.

2. **Stuffed Mushrooms**: Fill mushroom caps with a mixture of low-fat cream cheese, herbs, and spices for a savory and satisfying appetizer. Bake until the mushrooms are tender and the filling is golden brown for a flavorful bite-sized treat.

3. **Caprese Skewers**: Thread cherry tomatoes, fresh mozzarella balls, and basil leaves onto skewers for a classic Italian appetizer that's low in potassium and high in flavor. Drizzle with a balsamic glaze or reduction for added sweetness and depth of flavor.

4. **Cucumber Canapés**: Slice cucumbers into rounds and top with a dollop of low-sodium cream cheese or Greek yogurt, a slice of smoked salmon or turkey, and a sprinkle of fresh dill or chives for an elegant and refreshing appetizer.

5. **Deviled Eggs**: Prepare deviled eggs with a filling made from mashed hard-boiled egg yolks, low-fat mayonnaise, Dijon mustard, and a dash of paprika for added flavor. Garnish with fresh herbs or sliced green onions for a colorful and tasty appetizer option.

6. **Shrimp Cocktail**: Serve chilled shrimp with a tangy cocktail sauce made from low-sodium ketchup, horseradish, lemon

juice, and Worcestershire sauce for a classic seafood appetizer that's low in potassium and high in protein.

7. **Cucumber Sushi Rolls**: Roll thinly sliced cucumber around fillings like crab salad, avocado, or smoked salmon for a light and refreshing take on sushi. Serve with soy sauce or a low-sodium tamari for dipping.

8. **Bruschetta**: Top toasted whole grain baguette slices with a mixture of diced tomatoes, garlic, basil, olive oil, and balsamic vinegar for a flavorful and kidney-friendly appetizer option. Sprinkle with a pinch of salt-free Italian seasoning for added flavor.

Homemade Salsas and Dips

Salsas and dips are versatile accompaniments that can be served with a variety of snacks and appetizers. By making your own salsas and dips at home using kidney-friendly ingredients, you can control the sodium and potassium content and customize the flavors to suit your preferences. Here are some homemade salsa and dip ideas for individuals following a renal diet:

1. **Pico de Gallo**: Combine diced tomatoes, onions, jalapeños, cilantro, lime juice, and a pinch of salt for a fresh and flavorful salsa that's perfect for dipping chips or topping grilled meats and seafood.

2. **Guacamole**: Mash ripe avocados with diced onions, tomatoes, cilantro, lime juice, and a dash of cumin for a creamy and delicious dip that's rich in heart-healthy fats and low in sodium.

3. **Black Bean Salsa**: Mix canned black beans with diced tomatoes, onions, bell peppers, corn, cilantro, lime juice, and a sprinkle of chili powder for a protein-packed salsa that's perfect for scooping with tortilla chips or serving as a side dish.

4. **Greek Yogurt Dip**: Combine low-fat Greek yogurt with minced garlic, chopped dill, lemon juice, and a pinch of salt for a tangy and refreshing dip that pairs well with raw vegetables or whole grain crackers.

5. **Hummus**: Blend cooked chickpeas with tahini, lemon juice, garlic, olive oil, and a pinch of cumin for a creamy and nutritious dip that's high in protein and fiber. Serve with sliced vegetables or pita bread for dipping.

6. **Spinach Dip**: Mix thawed frozen spinach with low-fat sour cream, Greek yogurt, minced garlic, chopped scallions, and a sprinkle of grated Parmesan cheese for a creamy and flavorful dip that's perfect for parties or gatherings.

7. **Salsa Verde**: Blend tomatillos, jalapeños, onions, garlic, cilantro, lime juice, and a pinch of salt for a tangy and slightly

spicy salsa that's great for dipping tortilla chips or spooning over grilled meats and seafood.

8. **Tzatziki**: Combine grated cucumber, minced garlic, chopped dill, lemon juice, and Greek yogurt for a refreshing and tangy dip that's perfect for serving with grilled meats, pita bread, or raw vegetables.

By incorporating these snacks, appetizers, and homemade salsas and dips into your renal diet, you can enjoy flavorful and satisfying options that support your kidney health and overall well-being. Remember to consult with a healthcare provider or registered dietitian for personalized guidance and recommendations tailored to your individual dietary needs and preferences.

CHAPTER EIGHT

Side Dishes and Accompaniments

Side dishes and accompaniments play a crucial role in rounding out a meal and adding variety and texture to the plate. For individuals following a renal diet, choosing side dishes that are low in phosphorus, potassium, and sodium is essential to support kidney health. Here are some ideas for kidney-friendly side dishes and accompaniments:

Low-Phosphorus Vegetable Sides

Vegetables are a nutritious and versatile component of any meal, providing essential vitamins, minerals, and fiber. For individuals with kidney disease, choosing vegetables that are low in phosphorus can help manage blood phosphorus levels and support overall kidney health. Here are some low-phosphorus vegetable side dish ideas:

1. **Steamed Asparagus**: Steam fresh asparagus spears until tender-crisp, then season with a squeeze of lemon juice and a sprinkle of chopped fresh herbs such as parsley or dill.

2. **Roasted Brussels Sprouts**: Toss halved Brussels sprouts with olive oil, minced garlic, and a pinch of salt, then roast in the oven until caramelized and tender.

3. **Sautéed Spinach**: Sauté fresh spinach leaves with minced garlic and a drizzle of olive oil until wilted, then finish with a splash of lemon juice for brightness.

4. **Grilled Zucchini**: Slice zucchini into thin strips, brush with olive oil, and grill until tender and lightly charred. Sprinkle with grated Parmesan cheese for extra flavor.

5. **Braised Kale**: Braise kale leaves in low-sodium vegetable broth with diced onions and garlic until tender, then season with a pinch of red pepper flakes for heat.

6. **Stir-Fried Bok Choy**: Stir-fry bok choy with ginger, garlic, and a splash of low-sodium soy sauce until crisp-tender, then garnish with sesame seeds for crunch.

7. **Cauliflower Mash**: Steam cauliflower florets until soft, then mash with a potato masher until smooth. Season with salt, pepper, and a dollop of low-fat sour cream for creaminess.

8. **Green Bean Almondine**: Blanch green beans until crisp-tender, then toss with toasted slivered almonds and a drizzle of olive oil for a simple and elegant side dish.

Grain and Pasta Alternatives

Grains and pasta are staple ingredients that can be easily incorporated into meals as side dishes or main components. For individuals with kidney disease, choosing grain and pasta alternatives that are lower in phosphorus and potassium can help support kidney health. Here are some kidney-friendly grain and pasta alternatives:

1. **Quinoa**: Cook quinoa according to package instructions and fluff with a fork. Serve as a nutritious and protein-rich alternative to rice or pasta.

2. **Barley**: Simmer barley in low-sodium vegetable broth until tender, then use it as a base for salads, soups, or pilafs for added texture and flavor.

3. **Bulgur**: Soak bulgur in hot water until tender, then use it as a base for tabbouleh salad or as a stuffing for peppers or mushrooms.

4. **Brown Rice Pasta**: Substitute brown rice pasta for traditional wheat pasta in your favorite pasta dishes for a gluten-free and kidney-friendly option.

5. **Spaghetti Squash**: Roast spaghetti squash in the oven until tender, then scrape the flesh with a fork to create long strands that resemble spaghetti. Serve with marinara sauce or pesto for a low-carb alternative to pasta.

6. **Sorghum**: Cook sorghum in water or broth until tender, then use it as a base for grain bowls, salads, or pilafs for added nutrition and texture.

7. **Farro**: Cook farro in simmering water until tender, then use it as a base for grain salads, risottos, or soups for a hearty and nutritious option.

8. **Millet**: Toast millet in a dry skillet until fragrant, then simmer in water or broth until fluffy and tender. Serve as a side dish or use it as a base for breakfast porridge or stuffed peppers.

Renal-Friendly Potato and Rice Dishes

Potatoes and rice are classic side dishes that can be enjoyed in a variety of ways to complement a wide range of meals. For individuals with kidney disease, choosing renal-friendly potato and rice dishes that are lower in potassium and phosphorus can help support kidney health. Here are some ideas for kidney-friendly potato and rice dishes:

1. **Oven-Roasted Potatoes**: Toss diced potatoes with olive oil, garlic powder, and dried herbs such as rosemary or thyme. Roast in the oven until golden brown and crispy for a flavorful and satisfying side dish.

2. **Mashed Cauliflower**: Steam cauliflower florets until soft, then mash with a potato masher until smooth. Season with

salt, pepper, and a dollop of low-fat sour cream for a creamy and nutritious alternative to mashed potatoes.

3. **Potato Salad**: Boil diced potatoes until tender, then toss with diced celery, red onion, and a tangy dressing made from low-fat mayonnaise, Dijon mustard, and apple cider vinegar. Garnish with chopped fresh parsley for freshness.

4. **Brown Rice Pilaf**: Sauté diced onions and garlic in olive oil until soft, then add brown rice and toast until lightly golden. Add low-sodium vegetable broth and simmer until the rice is tender and fluffy. Stir in chopped nuts, dried fruit, and herbs for added flavor and texture.

5. **Hasselback Potatoes**: Make thin slices in whole potatoes without cutting all the way through, then brush with olive oil and sprinkle with salt, pepper, and dried herbs. Roast in the oven until crispy and golden brown for an elegant and visually appealing side dish.

6. **Wild Rice Salad**: Cook wild rice according to package instructions, then toss with diced bell peppers, green onions, dried cranberries, and a zesty vinaigrette made from olive oil, lemon juice, and Dijon mustard. Serve chilled for a refreshing and nutritious side dish.

7. **Potato Leek Soup**: Sauté sliced leeks in olive oil until soft, then add diced potatoes and low-sodium vegetable broth.

Simmer until the potatoes are tender, then puree until smooth. Season with salt, pepper, and a splash of low-fat milk for creaminess.

8. **Herbed Rice Pilaf**: Cook white or brown rice in low-sodium vegetable broth until tender, then stir in chopped fresh herbs such as parsley, dill, and chives. Fluff with a fork and serve as a flavorful and aromatic side dish.

By incorporating these side dishes and accompaniments into your renal diet, you can enjoy a variety of delicious and satisfying options that support kidney health and overall well-being. Remember to consult with a healthcare provider or registered dietitian for personalized guidance and recommendations tailored to your individual dietary needs and preferences.

CHAPTER NINE

Desserts and Treats

Desserts and treats are a delightful way to end a meal or indulge in a sweet snack. For individuals following a renal diet, it's essential to choose desserts that are not only delicious but also kidney-friendly, taking into account restrictions on potassium, phosphorus, and sugar. Here are some ideas for desserts and treats tailored to renal diets:

Fruit-Based Desserts with Low Potassium

Fruit-based desserts offer natural sweetness and are a nutritious option for satisfying your sweet tooth while adhering to a renal diet. By choosing fruits that are lower in potassium and pairing them with complementary flavors, you can create delicious desserts that support kidney health. Here are some fruit-based dessert ideas with low potassium:

1. **Berry Parfait**: Layer fresh berries such as strawberries, blueberries, and raspberries with low-fat yogurt or Greek yogurt in a glass or bowl. Top with a sprinkle of granola or chopped nuts for added texture and crunch.

2. **Grilled Fruit Kabobs**: Skewer chunks of low-potassium fruits such as pineapple, peaches, and mango onto wooden skewers and grill until caramelized. Serve with a drizzle of honey or a sprinkle of cinnamon for a simple and flavorful dessert.

3. **Watermelon Sorbet**: Blend chunks of seedless watermelon until smooth, then freeze in an ice cream maker until firm. Serve scoops of watermelon sorbet in chilled bowls for a refreshing and low-calorie dessert option.

4. **Baked Apples**: Core apples and fill the center with a mixture of chopped nuts, dried fruit, cinnamon, and a drizzle of honey. Bake until the apples are tender and caramelized for a warm and comforting dessert.

5. **Frozen Banana Bites**: Slice bananas into rounds and dip them in melted dark chocolate. Place the chocolate-dipped banana slices on a parchment-lined baking sheet and freeze until firm for a decadent and potassium-friendly treat.

6. **Mango Coconut Popsicles**: Blend ripe mangoes with coconut milk and a splash of lime juice until smooth, then pour the mixture into popsicle molds and freeze until set. Enjoy creamy and tropical popsicles with a fraction of the potassium found in traditional dairy-based desserts.

7. **Mixed Fruit Salad**: Toss together a variety of low-potassium fruits such as melon cubes, kiwi slices, and grapes in a bowl. Drizzle with a mixture of honey and lime juice for a refreshing and naturally sweet dessert option.

8. **Peach Cobbler Cups**: Layer sliced peaches in individual ramekins and top with a mixture of oats, almond flour, cinnamon, and a drizzle of maple syrup. Bake until the topping is golden brown and crispy for a comforting and portion-controlled dessert.

Decadent Renal-Friendly Desserts

Indulgent desserts can still be enjoyed on a renal diet with some modifications to traditional recipes. By using kidney-friendly ingredients and reducing the amounts of potassium, phosphorus, and sugar, you can create decadent desserts that satisfy your cravings without compromising your kidney health. Here are some ideas for renal-friendly indulgences:

1. **Chocolate Avocado Mousse**: Blend ripe avocados with cocoa powder, vanilla extract, and a sweetener of your choice (such as honey or maple syrup) until smooth and creamy. Chill the mixture in the refrigerator until firm for a rich and velvety chocolate mousse.

2. **Almond Flour Brownies**: Substitute almond flour for all-purpose flour in your favorite brownie recipe to reduce the phosphorus content. Add chopped nuts or dark chocolate

chunks for extra flavor and texture without increasing potassium levels.

3. **Coconut Chia Pudding**: Mix chia seeds with coconut milk and a touch of sweetener, then refrigerate until thickened. Serve the coconut chia pudding topped with fresh berries or toasted coconut flakes for a creamy and indulgent dessert.

4. **Peanut Butter Banana Nice Cream**: Blend frozen bananas with peanut butter and a splash of almond milk until smooth and creamy. Serve the peanut butter banana nice cream in bowls with a drizzle of sugar-free chocolate sauce for a guilt-free treat.

5. **Lemon Cheesecake Bars**: Make a kidney-friendly version of cheesecake by using low-fat cream cheese, Greek yogurt, and a graham cracker crust made with crushed low-sodium crackers. Add lemon zest and juice for a tangy and refreshing twist.

6. **Pumpkin Spice Bread Pudding**: Use whole grain bread and low-fat milk in your favorite bread pudding recipe to reduce phosphorus and sodium levels. Add canned pumpkin puree, cinnamon, nutmeg, and cloves for a festive and flavorful dessert.

7. **Vanilla Bean Panna Cotta**: Make a creamy and indulgent panna cotta using low-fat milk, gelatin, and vanilla bean

paste. Serve the vanilla bean panna cotta topped with fresh berries or a fruit compote for a sophisticated and kidney-friendly dessert option.

8. **Cinnamon Roll Oatmeal Cookies**: Bake oatmeal cookies flavored with cinnamon, vanilla extract, and a touch of maple syrup for sweetness. Add raisins or chopped nuts for extra flavor and texture without increasing phosphorus levels.

Sugar-Free and Low-Phosphorus Treats

For individuals with kidney disease who need to limit their sugar and phosphorus intake, there are plenty of delicious treats that can be enjoyed without compromising kidney health. By using alternative sweeteners and carefully selecting ingredients, you can satisfy your sweet cravings while managing your dietary restrictions. Here are some ideas for sugar-free and low-phosphorus treats:

1. **Sugar-Free Gelatin Cups**: Make sugar-free gelatin cups using sugar-free gelatin mix and water. Add diced fruit such as berries or peaches for extra flavor and texture without adding sugar or phosphorus.

2. **Homemade Trail Mix**: Create a custom trail mix using unsalted nuts, seeds, and dried fruit. Mix together almonds, walnuts, pumpkin seeds, and unsweetened dried cranberries or apricots for a satisfying and portable snack.

3. **Chocolate-Dipped Strawberries**: Dip fresh strawberries in melted dark chocolate sweetened with a sugar substitute such as stevia or erythritol. Allow the chocolate-dipped strawberries to set in the refrigerator until firm for a decadent and kidney-friendly treat.

4. **Baked Cinnamon Apple Chips**: Slice apples thinly and toss them with cinnamon and a touch of sweetener, then bake in the oven until crisp. Enjoy baked cinnamon apple chips as a crunchy and low-calorie snack option.

5. **Sugar-Free Popsicles**: Make homemade popsicles using sugar-free fruit juice or herbal tea sweetened with a sugar substitute. Pour the mixture into popsicle molds and freeze until set for a refreshing and guilt-free treat.

6. **Low-Phosphorus Rice Cakes**: Top rice cakes with unsweetened almond butter or peanut butter and sliced bananas or apples for a satisfying and low-phosphorus snack option. Sprinkle with cinnamon for added flavor without adding sugar.

7. **Chia Seed Energy Bites**: Mix chia seeds with nut butter, rolled oats, and a touch of honey or maple syrup for sweetness. Roll the mixture into bite-sized balls and refrigerate until firm for a nutritious and portable snack.

8. **Greek Yogurt Bark**: Spread low-fat Greek yogurt onto a parchment-lined baking sheet and swirl in sugar-free fruit jam or puree. Freeze until firm, then break into pieces for a creamy and refreshing treat.

By incorporating these desserts and treats into your renal diet, you can satisfy your sweet cravings while supporting kidney health and overall well-being. Remember to enjoy these indulgences in moderation and consult with a healthcare provider or registered dietitian for personalized guidance and recommendations tailored to your individual dietary needs and preferences.

CHAPTER TEN

Beverages and Drinks

Beverages and drinks play a significant role in maintaining hydration and overall well-being, especially for individuals with kidney health concerns. Proper hydration is crucial for supporting kidney function and overall health, while choosing the right beverages can help manage potassium intake and provide refreshing options. Here are some ideas for beverages and drinks tailored to renal health:

Hydration Tips for Renal Health

Staying hydrated is essential for kidney health, as adequate fluid intake helps support kidney function and maintain overall well-being. Individuals with kidney disease may have specific hydration needs depending on their condition and treatment plan. Here are some hydration tips for renal health:

1. **Drink Plenty of Water**: Water is the best choice for staying hydrated, as it is free of calories, additives, and potential kidney-stressing compounds. Aim to drink at least eight

glasses of water per day, or more if recommended by your healthcare provider.

2. **Monitor Urine Output**: Pay attention to your urine output as a gauge of hydration. Clear or pale yellow urine indicates adequate hydration, while dark-colored urine may signal dehydration and the need to drink more fluids.

3. **Spread Fluid Intake Throughout the Day**: Drink fluids steadily throughout the day rather than consuming large amounts at once. Sipping water or other hydrating beverages regularly can help maintain hydration levels and support kidney function.

4. **Limit High-Sugar Beverages**: Avoid sugary drinks such as soda, fruit juice, and sweetened teas, as they can contribute to excessive calorie intake and may exacerbate kidney health issues. Opt for sugar-free or low-sugar alternatives whenever possible.

5. **Watch Your Sodium Intake**: Be mindful of sodium intake, as excessive sodium consumption can lead to fluid retention and exacerbate kidney problems. Choose low-sodium beverages and avoid adding salt to your drinks.

6. **Consider Electrolyte Balance**: If you have kidney disease, electrolyte imbalances may occur, affecting hydration levels. Discuss with your healthcare provider or dietitian about

appropriate electrolyte intake and consider incorporating electrolyte-balanced beverages as needed.

7. **Monitor Fluid Restrictions**: Some individuals with advanced kidney disease may need to restrict fluid intake to manage fluid overload and prevent complications. Follow your healthcare provider's recommendations regarding fluid intake limits.

8. **Choose Kidney-Friendly Beverages**: Opt for kidney-friendly beverages such as herbal teas, infused water, and homemade fruit juices to stay hydrated while managing kidney health. These options are low in potassium and phosphorus, making them suitable for renal diets.

Low-Potassium Drink Options

For individuals with kidney disease, managing potassium intake is crucial to prevent hyperkalemia (high potassium levels) and maintain proper electrolyte balance. Choosing low-potassium drink options can help support kidney health while providing refreshing and hydrating beverages. Here are some low-potassium drink options:

1. **Herbal Teas**: Enjoy herbal teas such as chamomile, peppermint, or rooibos as low-potassium alternatives to traditional tea and coffee. These caffeine-free options are hydrating and offer various flavors to suit your preferences.

2. **Clear Broth**: Sip on clear broth made from low-sodium bouillon cubes or homemade stock as a warm and savory beverage option. Clear broths are low in potassium and can help replenish fluids and electrolytes.

3. **Coconut Water**: Coconut water is a natural source of electrolytes, including potassium, but it typically contains less potassium compared to fruit juices. Choose unsweetened coconut water and consume in moderation to avoid excessive potassium intake.

4. **Sparkling Water**: Enjoy plain or flavored sparkling water as a refreshing and hydrating drink option that is free of calories, sugar, and potassium. Add a splash of lemon or lime juice for extra flavor without increasing potassium levels.

5. **Lemonade (made with low-potassium sweeteners)**: Prepare homemade lemonade using low-potassium sweeteners such as stevia or erythritol instead of traditional sugar. Squeeze fresh lemon juice and dilute with water for a tangy and hydrating beverage.

6. **Apple Juice (diluted with water)**: Dilute apple juice with water to reduce its potassium concentration while still enjoying its natural sweetness. Choose unsweetened apple juice and mix with equal parts water for a refreshing and low-potassium drink option.

7. **Infused Water**: Infuse water with slices of cucumber, mint leaves, citrus fruits, or berries for added flavor and hydration without increasing potassium levels. Experiment with different combinations to create your favorite infused water recipes.

8. **Iced Herbal Tea**: Brew herbal teas such as hibiscus, ginger, or lemongrass and chill them in the refrigerator for a refreshing iced beverage option. Add a few ice cubes and a slice of lemon or lime for extra refreshment.

Homemade Infusions and Refreshing Beverages

Creating homemade infusions and refreshing beverages allows you to customize flavors while avoiding additives and excessive sugar or potassium content. By using fresh ingredients and natural flavorings, you can enjoy hydrating drinks that support kidney health. Here are some ideas for homemade infusions and refreshing beverages:

1. **Cucumber Mint Infused Water**: Slice cucumbers and fresh mint leaves and place them in a pitcher of water. Allow the flavors to infuse for a few hours in the refrigerator before serving over ice for a crisp and refreshing drink.

2. **Ginger Lemonade**: Brew ginger tea by steeping fresh ginger slices in hot water, then let it cool to room temperature. Add freshly squeezed lemon juice and a touch of honey or stevia

for sweetness, then chill in the refrigerator before serving over ice.

3. **Berry Basil Sparkler**: Blend mixed berries (such as strawberries, blueberries, and raspberries) with fresh basil leaves and a splash of water until smooth. Strain the mixture to remove seeds, then pour over sparkling water for a vibrant and fizzy drink.

4. **Pineapple Coconut Cooler**: Blend fresh pineapple chunks with coconut water and ice until smooth and frothy. Serve the pineapple coconut cooler in chilled glasses garnished with a wedge of pineapple for a tropical and hydrating treat.

5. **Watermelon Mint Agua Fresca**: Puree seedless watermelon chunks with fresh mint leaves and a squeeze of lime juice until smooth. Strain the mixture to remove pulp, then pour over ice for a cooling and revitalizing agua fresca.

6. **Citrus Herb Infused Iced Tea**: Brew your favorite herbal tea, such as chamomile or lemongrass, and let it cool to room temperature. Add citrus slices (such as lemon, lime, and orange) and fresh herbs (such as basil or thyme) before chilling in the refrigerator and serving over ice.

7. **Cantaloupe Basil Refresher**: Blend ripe cantaloupe chunks with fresh basil leaves and a splash of coconut water until

smooth. Strain the mixture to remove pulp, then pour over ice for a light and aromatic refresher.

8. **Minty Green Tea Cooler**: Brew green tea bags in hot water, then let it cool to room temperature. Add fresh mint leaves and a squeeze of lemon juice, then chill in the refrigerator before serving over ice for a revitalizing and antioxidant-rich drink.

By incorporating these hydration tips, low-potassium drink options, and homemade infusions and refreshing beverages into your routine, you can stay hydrated while supporting kidney health and enjoying flavorful and refreshing drinks. Remember to consult with a healthcare provider or registered dietitian for personalized guidance and recommendations tailored to your individual dietary needs and preferences.

CHAPTER ELEVEN

RENAL DIETS AND THEIR PREPARATION

Low Sodium Diet

Ingredients:

- Fresh vegetables (e.g., spinach, broccoli, carrots)
- Lean meats (e.g., chicken breast, turkey)
- Fresh fruits (e.g., apples, oranges, berries)
- Whole grains (e.g., brown rice, quinoa, whole wheat bread)
- Herbs and spices (e.g., garlic, basil, black pepper)
- Low-sodium condiments (e.g., low-sodium soy sauce, vinegar)
- Olive oil or other healthy cooking oils

Instructions:

1. Begin by washing and preparing your vegetables. Chop them into desired sizes.

2. Preheat a non-stick pan over medium heat and add a small amount of olive oil.

3. Add the lean meat to the pan and cook until browned on both sides.

4. Remove the meat from the pan and set it aside.

5. In the same pan, add the chopped vegetables and cook until tender.

6. Meanwhile, cook the whole grains according to package instructions.

7. Once the vegetables are tender, add the cooked meat back into the pan.

8. Season with herbs, spices, and low-sodium condiments to taste.

9. Serve the cooked vegetables and meat alongside the whole grains.

10. Enjoy your delicious low sodium meal!

DASH Diet (Dietary Approaches to Stop Hypertension)

Ingredients:

- Fresh vegetables (e.g., kale, spinach, bell peppers)

- Fresh fruits (e.g., bananas, oranges, strawberries)
- Lean proteins (e.g., chicken breast, fish, tofu)
- Whole grains (e.g., brown rice, whole wheat pasta, oats)
- Low-fat dairy products (e.g., skim milk, Greek yogurt)
- Nuts and seeds (e.g., almonds, walnuts, chia seeds)
- Herbs and spices (e.g., garlic, oregano, turmeric)

Instructions:

1. Wash and chop the vegetables and fruits as needed.
2. Preheat a non-stick skillet over medium heat.
3. Add a small amount of olive oil or cooking spray to the skillet.
4. Add the lean protein (chicken breast, fish, tofu) to the skillet and cook until done.
5. Meanwhile, cook the whole grains according to package instructions.
6. In a separate pan, lightly sauté the fresh vegetables until tender.
7. Once the protein and vegetables are cooked, portion them onto plates.
8. Serve alongside the cooked whole grains and fresh fruits.

9. Garnish with herbs and spices for added flavor.

10. Enjoy your nutritious DASH diet meal, designed to help manage hypertension and promote overall health!

Mediterranean Diet

Ingredients:

- Extra virgin olive oil
- Fresh vegetables (e.g., tomatoes, cucumbers, bell peppers)
- Leafy greens (e.g., spinach, kale, arugula)
- Whole grains (e.g., bulgur, farro, whole grain bread)
- Lean proteins (e.g., fish, chicken, legumes)
- Fresh fruits (e.g., grapes, oranges, figs)
- Nuts and seeds (e.g., almonds, walnuts, sunflower seeds)
- Herbs and spices (e.g., basil, oregano, garlic)
- Dairy products (e.g., Greek yogurt, feta cheese)

Instructions:

1. Begin by washing and preparing your vegetables and fruits.
2. Cook whole grains according to package instructions and set aside.

3. Heat a non-stick pan over medium heat and add a small amount of olive oil.

4. Season your choice of lean protein (fish, chicken) with herbs and spices and cook until done.

5. In a large salad bowl, combine leafy greens, chopped vegetables, and fruits.

6. Drizzle with extra virgin olive oil and toss gently to coat.

7. Add cooked whole grains and lean protein to the salad.

8. Sprinkle with nuts and seeds for extra crunch and nutrition.

9. Serve immediately and enjoy your Mediterranean-inspired meal!

Plant-Based Diet

Ingredients:

- Fresh vegetables (e.g., broccoli, cauliflower, carrots)
- Leafy greens (e.g., spinach, kale, Swiss chard)
- Whole grains (e.g., quinoa, brown rice, barley)
- Legumes (e.g., lentils, chickpeas, black beans)
- Fresh fruits (e.g., apples, bananas, berries)
- Nuts and seeds (e.g., almonds, chia seeds, flaxseeds)

- Plant-based proteins (e.g., tofu, tempeh, seitan)
- Herbs and spices (e.g., cilantro, cumin, turmeric)
- Healthy fats (e.g., avocado, olive oil, coconut oil)

Instructions:

1. Wash and chop your vegetables and fruits as needed.
2. Cook whole grains and legumes according to package instructions and set aside.
3. Preheat a non-stick skillet over medium heat.
4. Add a small amount of olive oil or cooking spray to the skillet.
5. Cook plant-based proteins (tofu, tempeh) until golden brown and crispy.
6. In a large bowl, combine cooked whole grains, legumes, and sautéed vegetables.
7. Add fresh fruits and leafy greens to the bowl.
8. Drizzle with a dressing made from olive oil, lemon juice, and your choice of herbs and spices.
9. Garnish with nuts and seeds for added texture and flavor.
10. Serve your plant-based meal and savor the delicious and nutritious flavors!

Low Potassium Diet

Ingredients:

- Low-potassium fruits (e.g., apples, berries, grapes)
- Low-potassium vegetables (e.g., cabbage, cauliflower, green beans)
- White bread or bread made with refined flour
- White rice or pasta made with refined flour
- Lean proteins (e.g., chicken breast, fish, egg whites)
- Cooking oils (e.g., olive oil, canola oil)
- Fresh herbs and spices (e.g., basil, parsley, thyme)
- Low-potassium dairy substitutes (e.g., rice milk, almond milk)
- Low-potassium snacks (e.g., rice cakes, unsalted crackers)

Instructions:

1. Wash and prepare low-potassium fruits and vegetables as needed.
2. Cook lean proteins such as chicken breast or fish using your preferred method.
3. Boil or steam low-potassium vegetables until tender.
4. Cook white rice or pasta according to package instructions.

5. Serve the cooked lean proteins, vegetables, and grains together as a meal.

6. Use olive oil or canola oil for cooking and seasoning.

7. Garnish with fresh herbs and spices for added flavor.

8. Substitute regular dairy with low-potassium alternatives like rice milk or almond milk.

9. Enjoy your low-potassium meal while adhering to dietary restrictions!

Low Phosphorus Diet

Ingredients:

- Low-phosphorus fruits (e.g., apples, cranberries, pineapple)
- Low-phosphorus vegetables (e.g., cabbage, cucumber, radishes)
- White bread or bread made with refined flour
- White rice or pasta made with refined flour
- Lean proteins (e.g., chicken breast, turkey, egg whites)
- Cooking oils (e.g., olive oil, canola oil)
- Fresh herbs and spices (e.g., garlic powder, onion powder, basil)

- Low-phosphorus dairy substitutes (e.g., almond milk, coconut milk)
- Low-phosphorus snacks (e.g., rice cakes, unsalted popcorn)

Instructions:

1. Wash and prepare low-phosphorus fruits and vegetables as needed.
2. Cook lean proteins such as chicken breast or turkey using your preferred method.
3. Boil or steam low-phosphorus vegetables until tender.
4. Cook white rice or pasta according to package instructions.
5. Serve the cooked lean proteins, vegetables, and grains together as a meal.
6. Use olive oil or canola oil for cooking and seasoning.
7. Season dishes with fresh herbs and spices for added flavor without added phosphorus.
8. Substitute regular dairy with low-phosphorus alternatives like almond milk or coconut milk.
9. Enjoy your low-phosphorus meal while adhering to dietary restrictions!

Low Protein Diet

Ingredients:

- Low-protein grains and starches (e.g., white bread, white rice, pasta)
- Low-protein fruits (e.g., apples, berries, peaches)
- Low-protein vegetables (e.g., lettuce, cucumbers, bell peppers)
- Healthy fats (e.g., olive oil, avocados, nuts)
- Low-protein dairy substitutes (e.g., almond milk, coconut milk)
- Eggs (in moderation)
- Fresh herbs and spices (e.g., basil, oregano, garlic powder)
- Low-protein snacks (e.g., rice cakes, unsalted popcorn)

Instructions:

1. Cook low-protein grains such as white rice or pasta according to package instructions.
2. Wash and prepare low-protein fruits and vegetables as needed.
3. Serve the cooked grains with a variety of fresh vegetables as a salad or side dish.

4. Use healthy fats like olive oil or avocado to add flavor to your dishes.

5. Incorporate low-protein dairy substitutes like almond milk or coconut milk into recipes or as beverages.

6. Include eggs in moderation as a source of protein.

7. Season dishes with fresh herbs and spices for added flavor.

8. Enjoy low-protein snacks such as rice cakes or unsalted popcorn when hunger strikes.

9. Follow these guidelines to create satisfying meals while adhering to a low-protein diet.

Paleo Diet

Ingredients:

- Lean meats (e.g., chicken breast, turkey, lean cuts of beef)
- Fish and seafood (e.g., salmon, tuna, shrimp)
- Eggs
- Fresh fruits (e.g., berries, apples, oranges)
- Fresh vegetables (e.g., broccoli, spinach, kale)
- Nuts and seeds (e.g., almonds, walnuts, chia seeds)
- Healthy fats (e.g., avocado, olive oil, coconut oil)

- Herbs and spices (e.g., garlic, basil, turmeric)
- Limited amounts of natural sweeteners (e.g., honey, maple syrup)

Instructions:

1. Cook lean meats, fish, or seafood using your preferred method (grilling, baking, sautéing).
2. Incorporate eggs into meals as desired.
3. Wash and enjoy fresh fruits and vegetables raw or lightly cooked.
4. Include nuts and seeds as snacks or toppings for salads and dishes.
5. Use healthy fats like avocado, olive oil, or coconut oil for cooking and dressing.
6. Season dishes with herbs and spices for added flavor.
7. Limit consumption of processed foods and refined sugars.
8. Experiment with paleo-friendly recipes to create a variety of satisfying meals.
9. Embrace the paleo lifestyle by focusing on whole, nutrient-dense foods while avoiding processed ingredients.

Ketogenic Diet

Ingredients:

- High-fat meats (e.g., bacon, fatty cuts of beef, chicken thighs with skin)
- Fatty fish (e.g., salmon, mackerel, sardines)
- Eggs
- Low-carb vegetables (e.g., spinach, kale, cauliflower, broccoli)
- High-fat dairy products (e.g., cheese, heavy cream, butter)
- Nuts and seeds (e.g., almonds, macadamia nuts, chia seeds)
- Avocados
- Healthy oils (e.g., coconut oil, olive oil, avocado oil)
- Low-carb sweeteners (e.g., stevia, erythritol)
- Herbs and spices (e.g., garlic powder, onion powder, paprika)

Instructions:

1. Choose high-fat meats and fatty fish for your main protein sources.
2. Cook meats and fish using healthy oils like coconut oil or olive oil.
3. Incorporate eggs into meals as desired.

4. Enjoy low-carb vegetables such as spinach, kale, cauliflower, and broccoli either raw or cooked in dishes.

5. Include high-fat dairy products like cheese, heavy cream, and butter in recipes and as toppings.

6. Snack on nuts and seeds or incorporate them into meals for added texture and flavor.

7. Add avocado to meals or enjoy it as a snack for healthy fats.

8. Use healthy oils for cooking and salad dressings.

9. Sweeten dishes with low-carb sweeteners like stevia or erythritol.

10. Season dishes with herbs and spices for added flavor without adding carbs.

11. Follow these guidelines to create satisfying meals while adhering to a ketogenic diet.

Flexitarian Diet

Ingredients:

- Plant-based proteins (e.g., tofu, tempeh, legumes)
- Whole grains (e.g., quinoa, brown rice, barley)
- Fresh fruits (e.g., apples, bananas, berries)
- Fresh vegetables (e.g., broccoli, carrots, bell peppers)

- Nuts and seeds (e.g., almonds, walnuts, flaxseeds)
- Dairy products (e.g., Greek yogurt, cottage cheese)
- Eggs
- Lean meats (optional, in small quantities)
- Fish and seafood (optional, in small quantities)
- Herbs and spices (e.g., basil, cilantro, cumin)

Instructions:

1. Incorporate plant-based proteins such as tofu, tempeh, and legumes into meals.
2. Cook whole grains like quinoa, brown rice, or barley as a base for dishes.
3. Enjoy a variety of fresh fruits and vegetables either raw or cooked in dishes.
4. Include nuts and seeds in meals or as snacks for added texture and nutrition.
5. Incorporate dairy products like Greek yogurt or cottage cheese into recipes or as snacks.
6. Use eggs as a versatile protein source in meals.
7. Optionally, include lean meats, fish, or seafood in small quantities if desired.

8. Season dishes with herbs and spices for added flavor without adding extra calories.

9. Experiment with different combinations of ingredients to create satisfying and nutritious meals.

10. Embrace the flexibility of the flexitarian diet by incorporating a variety of plant-based foods while still allowing for occasional animal products.

Weight Watchers (WW)

Ingredients:

- Lean proteins (e.g., skinless chicken breast, turkey breast, fish)
- Fresh vegetables (e.g., spinach, broccoli, bell peppers)
- Fresh fruits (e.g., apples, berries, oranges)
- Whole grains (e.g., brown rice, quinoa, whole wheat pasta)
- Low-fat dairy products (e.g., Greek yogurt, skim milk, cottage cheese)
- Eggs
- Legumes (e.g., lentils, chickpeas, black beans)
- Nuts and seeds (e.g., almonds, walnuts, chia seeds)
- Herbs and spices (e.g., garlic, basil, paprika)

- Healthy cooking oils (e.g., olive oil, avocado oil)

Instructions:

1. Choose lean proteins such as skinless chicken breast, turkey breast, or fish as the main focus of your meals.

2. Fill your plate with plenty of fresh vegetables like spinach, broccoli, and bell peppers.

3. Enjoy fresh fruits as snacks or desserts to satisfy your sweet cravings.

4. Incorporate whole grains like brown rice, quinoa, or whole wheat pasta into your meals for added fiber and nutrients.

5. Include low-fat dairy products like Greek yogurt, skim milk, or cottage cheese for calcium and protein.

6. Use eggs as a versatile protein source in meals or as a quick and easy breakfast option.

7. Add legumes such as lentils, chickpeas, or black beans to soups, salads, or stir-fries for added protein and fiber.

8. Enjoy nuts and seeds in moderation as a source of healthy fats and crunch in salads or as snacks.

9. Season dishes with herbs and spices for added flavor without extra calories.

10. Use healthy cooking oils like olive oil or avocado oil for sautéing or dressing salads.

11. Follow the WW program guidelines to track your food intake and stay within your daily SmartPoints allowance.

12. Enjoy delicious and satisfying meals while still reaching your weight loss or maintenance goals.

Ornish Diet

Ingredients:

- Whole grains (e.g., brown rice, quinoa, oats)
- Fresh vegetables (e.g., leafy greens, carrots, broccoli)
- Fresh fruits (e.g., apples, oranges, berries)
- Legumes (e.g., lentils, chickpeas, black beans)
- Soy products (e.g., tofu, tempeh, edamame)
- Non-fat dairy products (e.g., skim milk, non-fat yogurt)
- Fish (e.g., salmon, trout, sardines)
- Poultry (e.g., skinless chicken breast, turkey breast)
- Nuts and seeds (e.g., almonds, walnuts, flaxseeds)
- Herbs and spices (e.g., garlic, ginger, turmeric)
- Healthy fats (e.g., avocado, olive oil, flaxseed oil)

Instructions:

1. Base your meals around whole grains like brown rice, quinoa, or oats for sustained energy and fiber.

2. Fill your plate with a variety of fresh vegetables such as leafy greens, carrots, and broccoli for vitamins and minerals.

3. Enjoy fresh fruits as snacks or desserts to satisfy your sweet cravings.

4. Include legumes such as lentils, chickpeas, or black beans in soups, stews, or salads for plant-based protein and fiber.

5. Incorporate soy products like tofu, tempeh, or edamame into meals as meat alternatives.

6. Choose non-fat dairy products like skim milk or non-fat yogurt for calcium and protein.

7. Include fish such as salmon, trout, or sardines in your diet for heart-healthy omega-3 fatty acids.

8. Opt for skinless poultry like chicken breast or turkey breast as a lean protein source.

9. Enjoy nuts and seeds in moderation for healthy fats, vitamins, and minerals.

10. Season dishes with herbs and spices for added flavor without extra calories.

11. Use healthy fats like avocado, olive oil, or flaxseed oil for cooking or dressing salads.

12. Follow the Ornish Diet guidelines to create balanced and nutritious meals while promoting heart health and overall well-being.

Atkins Diet

Ingredients:

- Protein sources (e.g., beef, pork, poultry, fish, eggs)
- Low-carb vegetables (e.g., spinach, broccoli, cauliflower, zucchini)
- High-fat dairy products (e.g., cheese, butter, heavy cream)
- Nuts and seeds (e.g., almonds, walnuts, chia seeds)
- Healthy oils (e.g., olive oil, coconut oil, avocado oil)
- Low-carb fruits (e.g., berries, avocados, tomatoes)
- Herbs and spices (e.g., garlic, basil, paprika)
- Sugar substitutes (e.g., stevia, erythritol)

Instructions:

1. Choose protein sources such as beef, pork, poultry, fish, and eggs as the foundation of your meals.

2. Include plenty of low-carb vegetables like spinach, broccoli, cauliflower, and zucchini to add fiber and nutrients.

3. Incorporate high-fat dairy products like cheese, butter, and heavy cream for added flavor and satiety.

4. Enjoy nuts and seeds such as almonds, walnuts, and chia seeds as snacks or toppings for salads and dishes.

5. Use healthy oils like olive oil, coconut oil, or avocado oil for cooking and salad dressings.

6. Include low-carb fruits like berries, avocados, and tomatoes in moderation for added sweetness.

7. Season dishes with herbs and spices for added flavor without extra carbs.

8. Use sugar substitutes like stevia or erythritol to sweeten dishes and beverages without adding extra calories or carbs.

9. Follow the Atkins Diet guidelines to gradually increase your carb intake over time while monitoring your weight loss and overall health.

Zone Diet

Ingredients:

- Lean proteins (e.g., chicken breast, turkey, fish, egg whites)

- Low-glycemic carbohydrates (e.g., whole grains, fruits, vegetables)
- Healthy fats (e.g., olive oil, avocado, nuts)
- Fresh fruits (e.g., berries, apples, oranges)
- Fresh vegetables (e.g., spinach, kale, bell peppers)
- Nuts and seeds (e.g., almonds, walnuts, flaxseeds)
- Whole grains (e.g., quinoa, brown rice, barley)
- Non-starchy vegetables (e.g., broccoli, cauliflower, green beans)
- Herbs and spices (e.g., garlic, ginger, basil)

Instructions:

1. Choose lean proteins such as chicken breast, turkey, fish, and egg whites as the main focus of your meals.
2. Incorporate low-glycemic carbohydrates like whole grains, fruits, and vegetables to provide sustained energy and fiber.
3. Include healthy fats like olive oil, avocado, and nuts to add flavor and satiety to meals.
4. Enjoy fresh fruits such as berries, apples, and oranges as snacks or desserts.

5. Fill your plate with a variety of fresh vegetables like spinach, kale, and bell peppers for vitamins and minerals.

6. Snack on nuts and seeds like almonds, walnuts, and flaxseeds for added protein and healthy fats.

7. Incorporate whole grains such as quinoa, brown rice, and barley into meals for complex carbohydrates.

8. Include non-starchy vegetables such as broccoli, cauliflower, and green beans to add volume and nutrients to dishes.

9. Season dishes with herbs and spices for added flavor without extra calories or sodium.

10. Follow the Zone Diet guidelines to create balanced and nutritious meals while maintaining proper macronutrient ratios for optimal health and weight management.

Raw Food Diet

Ingredients:

- Fresh fruits (e.g., berries, apples, bananas)
- Fresh vegetables (e.g., leafy greens, cucumbers, bell peppers)
- Raw nuts and seeds (e.g., almonds, walnuts, sunflower seeds)

- Raw grains and pseudo-grains (e.g., quinoa, buckwheat, oats)
- Sprouts (e.g., alfalfa sprouts, mung bean sprouts)
- Raw nut butters (e.g., almond butter, cashew butter)
- Cold-pressed oils (e.g., olive oil, coconut oil, flaxseed oil)
- Raw dairy alternatives (e.g., almond milk, coconut yogurt)
- Raw honey or maple syrup (as sweeteners)
- Sea salt, herbs, and spices (for seasoning)

Instructions:

1. Incorporate a variety of fresh fruits into your diet, such as berries, apples, and bananas, either whole or blended into smoothies.
2. Include a variety of fresh vegetables, such as leafy greens, cucumbers, and bell peppers, either raw or lightly steamed or sautéed if desired.
3. Enjoy raw nuts and seeds, such as almonds, walnuts, and sunflower seeds, as snacks or added to salads and dishes for crunch and nutrition.
4. Experiment with raw grains and pseudo-grains, such as quinoa, buckwheat, and oats, soaked or sprouted for increased digestibility.

5. Incorporate sprouts, such as alfalfa sprouts or mung bean sprouts, into salads, wraps, or sandwiches for added texture and nutrients.

6. Use raw nut butters, such as almond butter or cashew butter, as spreads or dips for fruits and vegetables.

7. Include cold-pressed oils, such as olive oil, coconut oil, or flaxseed oil, in salad dressings or raw food recipes for healthy fats.

8. Choose raw dairy alternatives, such as almond milk or coconut yogurt, as substitutes for traditional dairy products.

9. Sweeten dishes naturally with raw honey or maple syrup, and season dishes with sea salt, herbs, and spices for added flavor.

10. Embrace the simplicity and freshness of raw foods while enjoying the health benefits they provide.

Vegan Diet

Ingredients:

- Fresh fruits (e.g., apples, bananas, oranges)
- Fresh vegetables (e.g., spinach, kale, carrots)
- Legumes (e.g., lentils, chickpeas, black beans)
- Whole grains (e.g., quinoa, brown rice, oats)

- Nuts and seeds (e.g., almonds, chia seeds, flaxseeds)
- Plant-based proteins (e.g., tofu, tempeh, seitan)
- Dairy alternatives (e.g., almond milk, soy yogurt)
- Healthy fats (e.g., avocados, olive oil, coconut oil)
- Herbs and spices (e.g., basil, cilantro, turmeric)
- Plant-based sweeteners (e.g., maple syrup, agave nectar)

Instructions:

1. Fill your diet with a variety of fresh fruits, such as apples, bananas, and oranges, for natural sweetness and vitamins.
2. Include a variety of fresh vegetables, such as spinach, kale, and carrots, in salads, stir-fries, or soups for fiber and nutrients.
3. Incorporate legumes, such as lentils, chickpeas, and black beans, into meals for plant-based protein and fiber.
4. Choose whole grains, such as quinoa, brown rice, and oats, as the base for dishes like grain bowls, salads, or stir-fries.
5. Enjoy nuts and seeds, such as almonds, chia seeds, and flaxseeds, as snacks or added to dishes for healthy fats and protein.
6. Include plant-based proteins, such as tofu, tempeh, and seitan, in meals as meat alternatives or sources of protein.

7. Use dairy alternatives, such as almond milk or soy yogurt, in place of traditional dairy products in recipes and as beverages.

8. Incorporate healthy fats, such as avocados, olive oil, and coconut oil, into meals for flavor and satiety.

9. Season dishes with herbs and spices, such as basil, cilantro, and turmeric, for added flavor and health benefits.

10. Sweeten dishes naturally with plant-based sweeteners, such as maple syrup or agave nectar, when needed.

11. Embrace the variety and abundance of plant-based foods while enjoying the health benefits of a vegan lifestyle.

Carnivore Diet

Ingredients:

- Various cuts of meat (e.g., beef, pork, poultry, lamb)
- Organ meats (e.g., liver, kidneys, heart)
- Fish and seafood (e.g., salmon, mackerel, shrimp)
- Eggs
- Bone broth
- Butter or other animal fats
- Salt and pepper (for seasoning)

Instructions:

1. Base your meals around various cuts of meat such as beef, pork, poultry, or lamb.
2. Include organ meats like liver, kidneys, and heart for added nutrients.
3. Incorporate fish and seafood such as salmon, mackerel, or shrimp for variety.
4. Enjoy eggs cooked in various ways as a source of protein and healthy fats.
5. Drink bone broth for hydration and added nutrients.
6. Use butter or other animal fats for cooking and flavoring dishes.
7. Season meals with salt and pepper to taste.
8. Follow the Carnivore Diet guidelines to restrict carbohydrates and focus on animal-based foods for nutrition.
9. Monitor your health and consult with a healthcare professional if necessary while following this diet plan.

Specific Carbohydrate Diet (SCD)

Ingredients:

- Fresh fruits (e.g., apples, bananas, berries)

- Fresh vegetables (e.g., spinach, carrots, zucchini)
- Lean proteins (e.g., chicken breast, fish, eggs)
- Nuts and seeds (e.g., almonds, cashews, pumpkin seeds)
- Natural sweeteners (e.g., honey, maple syrup)
- Healthy fats (e.g., olive oil, avocado, coconut oil)
- Homemade yogurt (fermented for at least 24 hours)
- Fresh herbs and spices (e.g., basil, oregano, turmeric)

Instructions:

1. Enjoy a variety of fresh fruits such as apples, bananas, and berries as snacks or desserts.
2. Incorporate a variety of fresh vegetables such as spinach, carrots, and zucchini into meals for vitamins and minerals.
3. Choose lean proteins such as chicken breast, fish, or eggs as the main focus of your meals.
4. Snack on nuts and seeds such as almonds, cashews, or pumpkin seeds for added protein and healthy fats.
5. Use natural sweeteners such as honey or maple syrup in moderation to sweeten dishes or beverages.
6. Include healthy fats like olive oil, avocado, or coconut oil in cooking and salad dressings.

7. Enjoy homemade yogurt that has been fermented for at least 24 hours for probiotics and gut health.

8. Season dishes with fresh herbs and spices such as basil, oregano, or turmeric for added flavor and health benefits.

9. Follow the Specific Carbohydrate Diet guidelines to eliminate complex carbohydrates and focus on easily digestible foods to manage digestive disorders such as Crohn's disease or ulcerative colitis.

10. Monitor your symptoms and consult with a healthcare professional if necessary while following this diet plan.

Anti-Inflammatory Diet

Ingredients:

- Fatty fish (e.g., salmon, mackerel, sardines)
- Leafy greens (e.g., spinach, kale, Swiss chard)
- Cruciferous vegetables (e.g., broccoli, cauliflower, Brussels sprouts)
- Berries (e.g., blueberries, strawberries, raspberries)
- Nuts and seeds (e.g., almonds, walnuts, flaxseeds)
- Healthy fats (e.g., olive oil, avocado, coconut oil)
- Whole grains (e.g., quinoa, brown rice, oats)

- Turmeric and ginger (as anti-inflammatory spices)
- Garlic and onions (for their anti-inflammatory properties)
- Green tea (for its antioxidant properties)

Instructions:

1. Incorporate fatty fish like salmon, mackerel, or sardines into your diet for omega-3 fatty acids.

2. Enjoy a variety of leafy greens such as spinach, kale, and Swiss chard for their anti-inflammatory properties.

3. Include cruciferous vegetables like broccoli, cauliflower, and Brussels sprouts, which contain compounds that help reduce inflammation.

4. Snack on berries such as blueberries, strawberries, and raspberries, which are rich in antioxidants and have anti-inflammatory effects.

5. Incorporate nuts and seeds like almonds, walnuts, and flaxseeds into meals or as snacks for their anti-inflammatory fats.

6. Use healthy fats such as olive oil, avocado, or coconut oil in cooking and salad dressings.

7. Choose whole grains like quinoa, brown rice, or oats over refined grains for their fiber and nutrients.

8. Use turmeric and ginger liberally in cooking or as supplements for their potent anti-inflammatory properties.

9. Include garlic and onions in dishes for their anti-inflammatory and immune-boosting effects.

10. Drink green tea regularly for its antioxidant properties, which can help reduce inflammation.

11. Follow these guidelines to create meals that promote overall health and reduce inflammation in the body.

Alkaline Diet

Ingredients:

- Fresh fruits (e.g., apples, bananas, watermelon)
- Fresh vegetables (e.g., leafy greens, broccoli, carrots)
- Nuts and seeds (e.g., almonds, pumpkin seeds, sunflower seeds)
- Legumes (e.g., lentils, chickpeas, black beans)
- Healthy fats (e.g., avocados, olive oil, flaxseed oil)
- Plant-based proteins (e.g., tofu, tempeh, seitan)
- Alkaline water
- Herbal teas (e.g., chamomile, peppermint, ginger)
- Plant-based milks (e.g., almond milk, coconut milk)

- Alkaline grains (e.g., quinoa, millet, amaranth)

Instructions:

1. Fill your diet with a variety of fresh fruits such as apples, bananas, and watermelon, which have alkalizing effects on the body.

2. Include fresh vegetables like leafy greens, broccoli, and carrots in meals to help maintain an alkaline balance.

3. Snack on nuts and seeds such as almonds, pumpkin seeds, and sunflower seeds for their alkaline-forming properties.

4. Incorporate legumes like lentils, chickpeas, and black beans into meals as plant-based protein sources.

5. Use healthy fats such as avocados, olive oil, and flaxseed oil in cooking and salad dressings to support an alkaline environment.

6. Choose plant-based proteins like tofu, tempeh, and seitan over animal proteins, as they tend to be more alkaline-forming.

7. Drink alkaline water throughout the day to help maintain proper hydration and support the body's pH balance.

8. Enjoy herbal teas such as chamomile, peppermint, or ginger, which have alkalizing effects on the body.

9. Use plant-based milks like almond milk or coconut milk as alternatives to dairy milk, which can be acidic.

10. Incorporate alkaline grains like quinoa, millet, and amaranth into meals for their nutrient content and alkalizing effects.

11. Follow these guidelines to create meals that promote an alkaline environment in the body and support overall health and well-being.

Intermittent Fasting

Ingredients (for meal examples within eating windows):

- Lean proteins (e.g., chicken breast, turkey, fish)
- Healthy fats (e.g., avocado, nuts, olive oil)
- Low-glycemic index carbohydrates (e.g., quinoa, sweet potatoes, beans)
- Leafy greens and vegetables (e.g., spinach, kale, broccoli)
- Berries and other low-sugar fruits (e.g., strawberries, blueberries, apples)
- Whole grains (e.g., brown rice, whole grain bread, oats)
- Water and other non-caloric beverages

Instructions:

1. Choose a fasting window that fits your schedule, such as 16:8 (fasting for 16 hours, eating within an 8-hour window) or alternate-day fasting.

2. During the fasting period, consume only non-caloric beverages such as water, herbal tea, or black coffee.

3. Break your fast with a balanced meal that includes lean protein, healthy fats, and low-glycemic index carbohydrates to help stabilize blood sugar levels.

4. For example, a meal could consist of grilled chicken breast, steamed broccoli, and quinoa.

5. Incorporate leafy greens and vegetables into your meals to boost fiber intake and promote satiety.

6. Include berries and other low-sugar fruits for added flavor and nutrients.

7. Snack on nuts or enjoy a small portion of avocado to increase healthy fat intake.

8. Stay hydrated throughout the day by drinking water or other non-caloric beverages.

9. Consider experimenting with different fasting protocols and meal timings to find what works best for your lifestyle and goals.

10. Listen to your body and adjust your fasting schedule and meal choices as needed.

Low Glycemic Index (GI) Diet

Ingredients:

- Non-starchy vegetables (e.g., leafy greens, broccoli, cauliflower)
- Berries and other low-sugar fruits (e.g., strawberries, raspberries, apples)
- Whole grains (e.g., quinoa, barley, bulgur)
- Legumes (e.g., lentils, chickpeas, black beans)
- Lean proteins (e.g., chicken breast, turkey, tofu)
- Healthy fats (e.g., avocado, olive oil, nuts)
- Herbs and spices (e.g., garlic, cinnamon, turmeric)
- Low-fat dairy products (e.g., Greek yogurt, skim milk)
- Water and other non-caloric beverages

Instructions:

1. Choose non-starchy vegetables such as leafy greens, broccoli, and cauliflower as the base of your meals.
2. Incorporate berries and other low-sugar fruits like strawberries and raspberries for added flavor and nutrients.

3. Opt for whole grains like quinoa, barley, or bulgur over refined grains to keep blood sugar levels stable.

4. Include legumes such as lentils, chickpeas, or black beans for plant-based protein and fiber.

5. Choose lean proteins such as chicken breast, turkey, or tofu to reduce saturated fat intake.

6. Use healthy fats like avocado, olive oil, or nuts in moderation to add flavor and satiety to meals.

7. Flavor dishes with herbs and spices such as garlic, cinnamon, or turmeric instead of salt or sugar.

8. Include low-fat dairy products like Greek yogurt or skim milk for calcium and protein.

9. Stay hydrated by drinking water or other non-caloric beverages throughout the day.

10. Monitor portion sizes and listen to your body's hunger and fullness cues to maintain a balanced and satisfying diet.

11. Follow these guidelines to create meals that prioritize foods with a low glycemic index, promoting stable blood sugar levels and overall health.

Blood Type Diet

Ingredients: *(Note: The Blood Type Diet suggests different foods based on an individual's blood type. Below are general recommendations for each blood type.)*

For Type O:

- Lean proteins (e.g., beef, lamb, fish)
- Vegetables (e.g., spinach, broccoli, kale)
- Fruits (e.g., berries, plums, figs)
- Nuts and seeds (e.g., walnuts, pumpkin seeds, flaxseeds)
- Beans and legumes (e.g., lentils, navy beans, black-eyed peas)
- Healthy fats (e.g., olive oil, avocado, coconut oil)

For Type A:

- Plant-based proteins (e.g., tofu, tempeh, legumes)
- Vegetables (e.g., spinach, broccoli, carrots)
- Fruits (e.g., berries, apples, grapes)
- Whole grains (e.g., quinoa, brown rice, oats)
- Nuts and seeds (e.g., almonds, chia seeds, hemp seeds)
- Healthy fats (e.g., olive oil, flaxseed oil, avocado)

For Type B:

- Balanced diet with a variety of foods including lean proteins, vegetables, fruits, and grains
- Emphasis on moderate amounts of dairy, eggs, and certain meats such as lamb, rabbit, and venison
- Avoidance of chicken, corn, wheat, peanuts, and sesame seeds

For Type AB:

- Combination of recommendations for Type A and Type B, focusing on a balanced diet with a variety of plant-based foods and moderate amounts of lean proteins

Instructions:

1. Determine your blood type and follow the corresponding dietary recommendations.
2. Incorporate recommended foods for your blood type into your meals and snacks.
3. Include a variety of nutrient-rich foods such as lean proteins, vegetables, fruits, whole grains, nuts, and seeds.
4. Avoid foods that are not recommended for your blood type, as they may not be well-tolerated.
5. Pay attention to how your body responds to different foods and adjust your diet accordingly.

6. Stay hydrated by drinking plenty of water throughout the day.
7. Consider consulting with a healthcare professional or registered dietitian for personalized guidance and support.

Japanese Diet

Ingredients:

- Fish and seafood (e.g., salmon, tuna, shrimp)
- Rice
- Vegetables (e.g., seaweed, daikon radish, bamboo shoots)
- Soy products (e.g., tofu, edamame, miso)
- Fermented foods (e.g., pickles, fermented soybeans)
- Green tea
- Fruit (e.g., citrus fruits, persimmons)
- Noodles (e.g., soba noodles, udon noodles)
- Lean meats (e.g., chicken, pork)
- Eggs

Instructions:

1. Base meals around fish and seafood, which are staples of the Japanese diet and rich in omega-3 fatty acids.

2. Include rice as a main carbohydrate source, often served with a variety of dishes.

3. Incorporate a wide range of vegetables such as seaweed, daikon radish, and bamboo shoots, either raw or cooked.

4. Enjoy soy products like tofu, edamame, and miso, which provide protein and additional nutrients.

5. Include fermented foods such as pickles and fermented soybeans for their probiotic benefits and unique flavors.

6. Drink green tea regularly, as it is a common beverage in Japan and has various health benefits.

7. Enjoy fruits such as citrus fruits and persimmons as snacks or desserts.

8. Incorporate noodles such as soba noodles or udon noodles into meals for variety.

9. Include lean meats like chicken and pork in moderation, often served as part of a larger dish.

10. Use eggs as a versatile protein source, enjoyed in various dishes from breakfast to dinner.

11. Follow the Japanese tradition of enjoying smaller portions and savoring each bite mindfully.

12. Embrace the balance and variety of foods in the Japanese diet, which emphasizes fresh, seasonal ingredients and culinary techniques that enhance flavor and nutrition.

Nordic Diet

Ingredients:

- Fatty fish (e.g., salmon, herring, mackerel)
- Whole grains (e.g., rye, barley, oats)
- Berries (e.g., lingonberries, blueberries, cloudberries)
- Root vegetables (e.g., potatoes, carrots, beets)
- Cruciferous vegetables (e.g., cabbage, broccoli, Brussels sprouts)
- Legumes (e.g., beans, lentils)
- Rapeseed oil (canola oil)
- Nuts and seeds (e.g., almonds, hazelnuts, flaxseeds)
- Dairy products (e.g., yogurt, cheese)
- Wild game (e.g., elk, reindeer)
- Herbs and spices (e.g., dill, parsley, cardamom)

Instructions:

1. Base meals around fatty fish such as salmon, herring, or mackerel, which are rich in omega-3 fatty acids.

2. Incorporate whole grains like rye, barley, and oats into meals for fiber and nutrients.

3. Enjoy a variety of berries such as lingonberries, blueberries, and cloudberries for their antioxidants and flavor.

4. Include root vegetables like potatoes, carrots, and beets in dishes for their sweetness and nutritional value.

5. Incorporate cruciferous vegetables such as cabbage, broccoli, and Brussels sprouts for their health benefits.

6. Include legumes like beans and lentils as plant-based protein sources.

7. Use rapeseed oil (canola oil) for cooking and salad dressings, as it is a common oil in Nordic cuisine.

8. Snack on nuts and seeds such as almonds, hazelnuts, and flaxseeds for added protein and healthy fats.

9. Enjoy dairy products like yogurt and cheese for calcium and probiotics.

10. Include wild game such as elk or reindeer if available, as they are lean sources of protein.

11. Season dishes with herbs and spices like dill, parsley, and cardamom for added flavor without extra calories.

12. Follow the Nordic Diet principles of emphasizing seasonal, locally sourced ingredients and traditional cooking methods for a balanced and nutritious approach to eating.

South Beach Diet

Ingredients:

- Lean proteins (e.g., chicken breast, turkey, fish)
- Non-starchy vegetables (e.g., spinach, broccoli, peppers)
- Whole grains (e.g., quinoa, brown rice, whole wheat bread)
- Healthy fats (e.g., olive oil, avocado, nuts)
- Low-fat dairy products (e.g., Greek yogurt, skim milk)
- Legumes (e.g., lentils, black beans)
- Berries (e.g., strawberries, raspberries, blueberries)
- Herbs and spices (e.g., garlic, basil, cumin)
- Eggs

Instructions:

1. Base meals around lean proteins such as chicken breast, turkey, or fish for satiety and muscle maintenance.

2. Incorporate non-starchy vegetables like spinach, broccoli, and peppers into meals for fiber and vitamins.

3. Choose whole grains like quinoa, brown rice, or whole wheat bread over refined grains for sustained energy.

4. Include healthy fats like olive oil, avocado, and nuts in moderation for heart health and satiety.

5. Enjoy low-fat dairy products like Greek yogurt and skim milk for calcium and protein.

6. Include legumes such as lentils and black beans as plant-based protein sources and to add texture to meals.

7. Incorporate berries such as strawberries, raspberries, and blueberries for their antioxidants and natural sweetness.

8. Flavor dishes with herbs and spices like garlic, basil, and cumin for added flavor without extra calories.

9. Include eggs in your diet for a versatile protein source that can be enjoyed at any meal.

10. Follow the South Beach Diet principles of focusing on lean proteins, healthy fats, and fiber-rich carbohydrates to promote weight loss and overall health.

Macrobiotic Diet

Ingredients:

- Whole grains (e.g., brown rice, quinoa, barley)
- Beans and legumes (e.g., adzuki beans, lentils, chickpeas)
- Sea vegetables (e.g., nori, kombu, wakame)
- Fresh vegetables (e.g., leafy greens, root vegetables, cruciferous vegetables)
- Fermented foods (e.g., miso, tempeh, sauerkraut)
- Seafood (e.g., salmon, mackerel, sardines)
- Seeds and nuts (e.g., sesame seeds, pumpkin seeds, almonds)
- Fruits (e.g., apples, pears, berries)
- Herbal teas (e.g., green tea, dandelion tea, ginger tea)
- Natural sweeteners (e.g., maple syrup, brown rice syrup)

Instructions:

1. Base meals around whole grains such as brown rice, quinoa, or barley, which provide energy and fiber.
2. Include beans and legumes like adzuki beans, lentils, or chickpeas for plant-based protein and fiber.
3. Incorporate sea vegetables such as nori, kombu, or wakame for their mineral content and umami flavor.

4. Enjoy a variety of fresh vegetables, including leafy greens, root vegetables, and cruciferous vegetables, for vitamins and antioxidants.

5. Include fermented foods like miso, tempeh, or sauerkraut for their probiotic benefits and digestive health.

6. Include seafood such as salmon, mackerel, or sardines for omega-3 fatty acids and additional protein.

7. Snack on seeds and nuts like sesame seeds, pumpkin seeds, or almonds for healthy fats and protein.

8. Enjoy fruits such as apples, pears, and berries as snacks or desserts, preferably in season and locally sourced.

9. Drink herbal teas like green tea, dandelion tea, or ginger tea for hydration and additional health benefits.

10. Use natural sweeteners like maple syrup or brown rice syrup in moderation to sweeten dishes or beverages.

11. Follow the principles of balance and moderation in food choices and cooking methods to promote overall health and well-being.

12. Pay attention to chewing food thoroughly and eating mindfully as part of the macrobiotic lifestyle.

Low FODMAP Diet

Ingredients:

- Low-FODMAP fruits (e.g., bananas, berries, grapes)
- Low-FODMAP vegetables (e.g., carrots, cucumber, spinach)
- Gluten-free grains (e.g., rice, quinoa, oats)
- Protein sources (e.g., chicken, turkey, fish)
- Lactose-free dairy products (e.g., lactose-free milk, hard cheeses)
- Nuts and seeds (e.g., almonds, sunflower seeds, pumpkin seeds)
- Low-FODMAP sweeteners (e.g., maple syrup, sugar)
- Herbs and spices (e.g., basil, oregano, turmeric)
- Oils (e.g., olive oil, coconut oil)
- Non-caffeinated beverages (e.g., water, herbal teas)

Instructions:

1. Choose low-FODMAP fruits such as bananas, berries, and grapes for snacks or desserts.
2. Incorporate low-FODMAP vegetables like carrots, cucumber, and spinach into meals for fiber and nutrients.
3. Opt for gluten-free grains like rice, quinoa, or oats to avoid FODMAP-containing wheat products.

4. Include protein sources such as chicken, turkey, or fish in meals for satiety and muscle maintenance.

5. Use lactose-free dairy products like lactose-free milk or hard cheeses if tolerated, or opt for dairy alternatives.

6. Snack on nuts and seeds such as almonds, sunflower seeds, or pumpkin seeds for added protein and healthy fats.

7. Sweeten dishes with low-FODMAP sweeteners like maple syrup or sugar instead of high-FODMAP options.

8. Flavor dishes with herbs and spices such as basil, oregano, or turmeric for added taste without FODMAPs.

9. Cook with oils like olive oil or coconut oil for healthy fats and flavor.

10. Stay hydrated with non-caffeinated beverages like water or herbal teas.

11. Follow the low-FODMAP diet guidelines strictly, avoiding high-FODMAP foods and gradually reintroducing foods to identify triggers.

12. Consult with a registered dietitian specializing in the low-FODMAP diet for personalized guidance and support.

THE END

www.ingramcontent.com/pod-product-compliance
Lightning Source LLC
Chambersburg PA
CBHW062218220526
45471CB00009B/3254